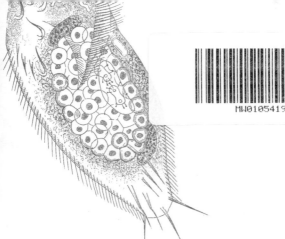

COLITIS & ME:
A STORY OF RECOVERY

BY RAMAN PRASAD

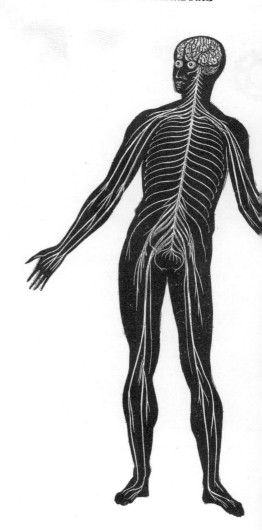

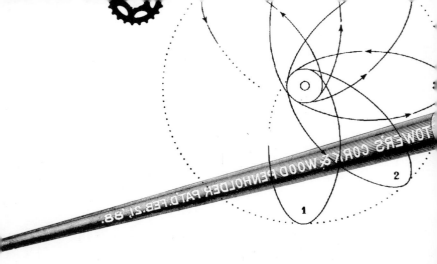

The author is not offering professional advice or services to the reader and suggestions in this book are in no way a substitute for medical evaluation and recommendations by a physician. The author and publisher are not liable or responsible for any direct loss or damage allegedly arising from any information or suggestion in this book or from the use of any treatments mentioned in this book. Before starting any kind of diet or medical treatment, it is advised that you consult your own health-care practitioner.

Copyright © 2002 Raman Prasad
All rights reserved.

Published by SCD Recipe LLC
www.scdrecipe.com

First Printing March 2003
Second Printing February 2004
Third Printing September 2005
Fourth Printing January 2007
Fifth Printing January 2010

ISBN 978-0-9727061-0-0

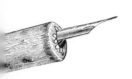

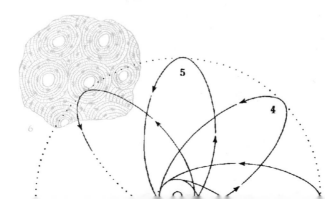

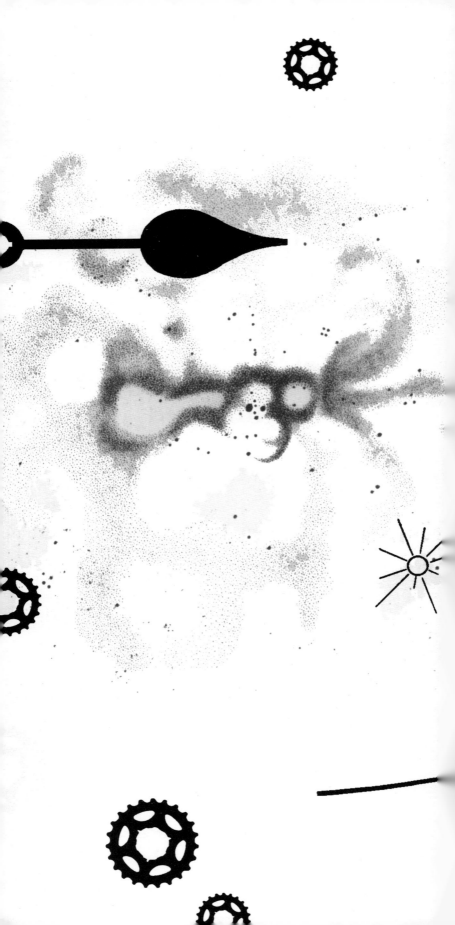

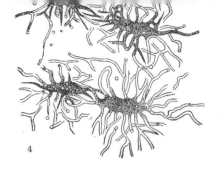

for:

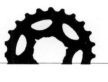

that spatula-wielding
garden-hoeing
sheetrock-repairing
trying-to-put-food-on-the-table
MOM

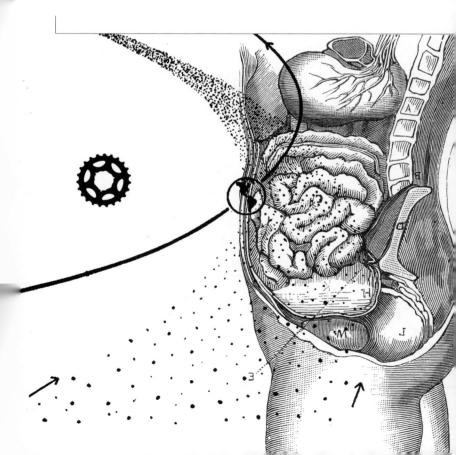

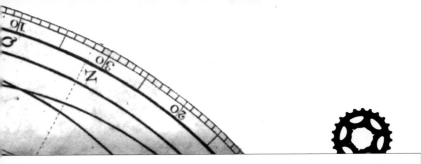

FOREWORD

by

Elaine Gottschall
Author of *Breaking the Vicious Cycle*

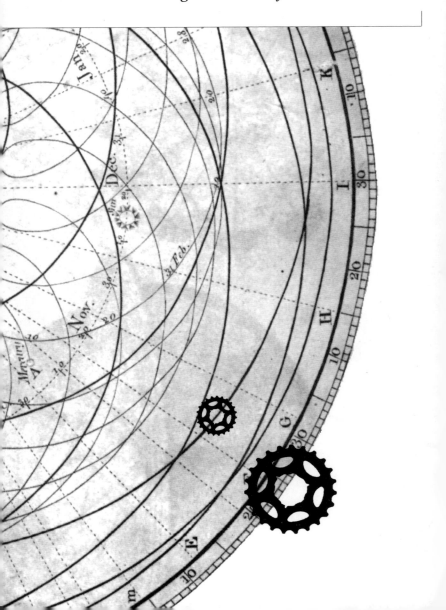

Raman Prasad's odyssey through the perils of ulcerative colitis is no less heroic than those of the original hero of the epic poem. His return to health, although not a product of modern medicine, is a product of good science.

Suffering with an illness such as ulcerative colitis has a few distinct and humiliating aspects. One is that because it happens below the belt the disease reduces one's dignity because the patient is constantly in fear. The patient with ulcerative colitis is secretive and suffers in silence, unlike the patient with a triple bypass who talks about his successes at gatherings, even to baring his chest to show his incision. Add to that, the hopelessness of being told his/her disease is incurable and the helplessness of being told he/she can do nothing about changing his/her diet to effect a cure.

But Raman and hundreds of others have found that what they are told is without foundation. The Specific Carbohydrate diet has brought many back to health because the doctor who developed the diet, Dr. Sidney Valentine Haas, was a scientist in the true word. He understood the world of intestinal bacteria and the effect of the modern diet on this world of microorganisms, and, subsequently, the immune system.

When Dr. Sidney Valentine Haas cured my child in the 1970's of ulcerative colitis, after three years of a perilous and painful experience such as Raman's, I knew I had found a workable solution. One cannot be quiet about such a miracle and, after years of academic study, years of watching the diet work its magic on hundreds, I wrote *Breaking the Vicious Cycle*.

We have a saying among us Specific Carbohydrate Dieters which reads, "We will reach one person at a time and will keep planting seeds." Raman's personal journey through ulcerative colitis recorded in this memoir *Colitis & Me: A Story of Recovery* is doing just that.

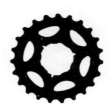

FEAR

Fear came from not knowing how you might feel each day. Finding the toilet bowl filled red with blood. The doctors probing you with the latest video imaging technology – giving you options of drugs or of ripping out the offending organs. Knowing that the drugs may not be effective in the long run and, at some point, that you may face either the knife or cancer, or both. You're not homeless, you're not eking out your life on the borderline of poverty. You're a decent person. You want to take care of yourself – to make choices, to pursue your own version of the American dream. It's there, you came damn far. But that road becomes a slippery highway: twisting, spilling you over the guardrail, hurtling you off the cliff. You're sick. You have a disease of unknown origin. You cannot modify your habits in order to control it. The doctors know that while your gut is hurting, it's harmful to eat raw vegetables, fruits, and nuts. In fact, they think it's best if you avoid these foods for the rest of your life. The best they can do is give you these pills which may or may not keep you in decent health for the months and years to come. They have found that stress is not the cause. But avoiding stress and doing exercise may make your road a bit less bumpy. Of course, there's no cure. You should expect that flare-ups will be a part of your life... like a bad tie given by an in-law that must be worn several times a year. You'll have to put on that tie, keep on grinning through the hard times.

Fear. Fear. Fear. Doctors have pronounced judgment upon you. If you go outside of what they say and try something different, well, the doctors may not be happy about it at all. They'll patiently tell you: listen, you'll have to live with it, why don't you get some more rest, take some more medication.

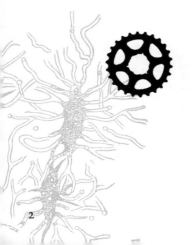

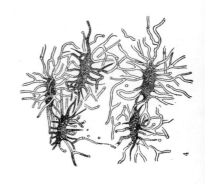

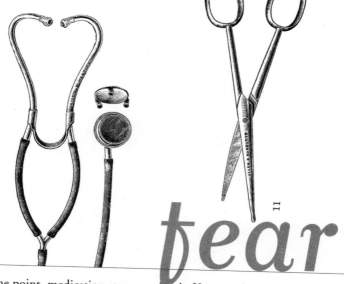

fear

At some point, medication stops cutting it. You may be sitting at work with your stomach twisting, slumping over your desk in pain. It may cause you to get pissed, to walk across your college campus with head up, face tight, back straight, not bending, using all of your concentration to fight the pain. When you walk, all your focus may go straight ahead. One step, two step. One, two. Head for the sign, the next lamp post. Tunnel vision. Focused. You must keep focused to keep going. The alternative is to bend to the pain, to go home, to lie in bed, to call up the doc, to call in sick, to drop out of life for a while. Each time you drop out, it's a little harder to move on: things have shifted, people change. You have to re-adjust, re-acquaint.

You may troop on, keep going despite the disease. You may be standing on the platform, waiting for the train. You're tense, because despite your neatly pressed clothes, things inside are twisted up. The pain's there, biting into you. You're trying to hold it back, but then it becomes unbearable. But you're still holding. The train's coming, chugging now, drowning out the conversations and footsteps around you. The door's open, people stream by you, funnel around you, bump into you. You watch from the platform as your train sets off without you. Tears come down, you can feel the blood in your pants, your body's broken, it's out of your control, you'll have to bring it back to the doc. Something will probably have to come out this time.

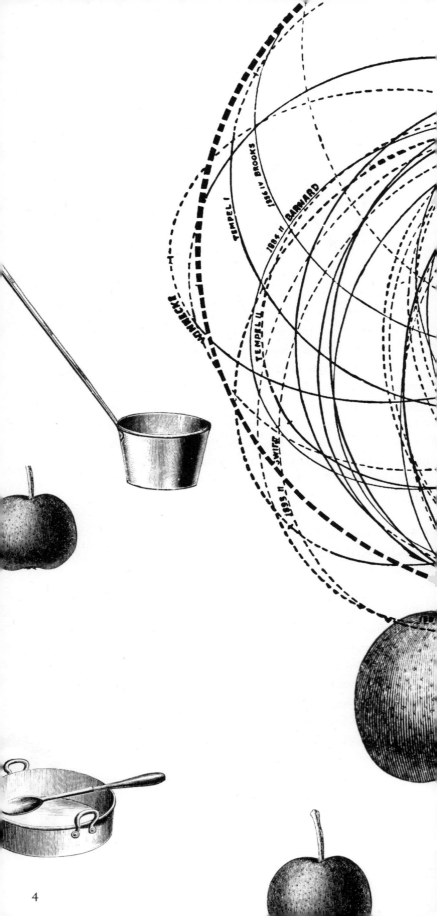

TEMPEL I

1886 IV BROOKS

1884 II BARNARD

WINNECKE

TEMPEL II

1889 II SWIFT

4

INTRODUCTION

Each morning, after my stretching, the day speeds up. For the 60th
consecutive working week, I grab two apples from the refrigerator
and hastily peel them, the skin piling up on a cutting board. I take
a knife, open the fridge again, cut a pat of butter and throw it into
the old cast iron frying pan given by my grandmother. I place the
pan over a low flame and begin the apple chopping. As the butter
melts, the bite-sized pieces of apple hit the pan and I run for the
shower. Returning to the kitchen in a towel, I turn off the stove.
In the bedroom I pull on pants and one of seven five-dollar T-shirts
– the same style I've been buying since high school. After putting
on a sweater, it's back to the kitchen: pull out an empty plastic container. Add generous dollops of yogurt, mix in the sautéed apples,
cap the container, and throw it into a nylon lunch bag. The lunch
bag goes into a backpack which I wear out the door, down the steps
of the brownstone, and past freshly painted wrought iron fences.
My legs feel loose. Wearing flat sneakers, I navigate past the stream
of people heading down into the subway tunnel. I walk past the
packed bagel shop, the tailor, the cobbler, the corner deli. Free of
the crowded block, I pass the restaurants of Smith Street. Even with
security shutters down, they hold happy memories of steak, tapas,
fish, salads, babaganoush! I check my watch and pick up my pace.
I see kids heading off to school, cyclists darting in and out of traffic.
I walk by an out of place surf shop sandwiched between neon-
windowed offices of bail bondsmen. Ahead looms the detention
center, a downtown jail undergoing never-ending renovations for
expansion.

Past the detention center and crowded parking lots, people head to
court: federal court and district court. Employees and lawyers check
their watches, adjust their ties. People with summonses in hand ask
directions. Court room veterans facing day-long waits amble in
unhurriedly. I wait for the stop lights at the intersection before the
Brooklyn bridge. A white line divides the bridge's walkway in half –
one side for bikers, the other for pedestrians. On the weekends, the
bridge becomes clogged. Bikers shout and wave, others blow whis-
tles as tourists walk on the wrong side. But it's Monday, no tourists.
Messengers shoot up and down the side. Runners, oblivious to the

traffic fumes, train hard. People go to work on bikes and on foot. The bridge waits ahead, gothic and gritty. Nearly one hundred twenty years old, it looks medieval. I see the flag blowing from the top. I'm feeling good, loose. Halfway across the bridge, I lean on the steel beam railing. Helicopters head toward the financial area. A tug-boat makes its way down river. I watch the water. I smile, picking up the pace again, thinking of the warm breakfast in my bag.

Life feels easy in my 29th year. But as I cross the second half of the bridge, descending into Manhattan, the little voice kicks in, remind-ing me that four years ago things were different. If not for a little luck, I might not have walked across this bridge – at least not with such ease. I had spent ages 17 through 24 with a bad gut, inflamma-tory bowel disease (IBD), ulcerative colitis. Thanks to a determined Canadian woman, a web site put up during the early internet days, and my mother who was able to pass on some of her cooking skills, I managed to find my way out of the doctors' offices and back into the world of the living.

I keep free of the ulcerative colitis by following a diet. Although the diet is not unknown, only a handful of doctors offer it as a treat-ment option to their IBD patients. Aside from these few, most doc-tors say that changing what you eat cannot be used to treat IBD. Or they say that studies must be done to prove it. However, they also admit that no one will fund studies. There's no profit in proving that diet can be used to help the million IBDers who take daily medication or need surgery and a steady supply of ostomy bags. Therefore, doctors present most patients with limited options.

In July 2000, I attended a family picnic and sat with the aunt of a 3rd cousin – whom I remember only as a toddler. The aunt explained that the cousin, Chris, was 12 years old, and that for the past six years has suffered from Crohn's disease. Each night he hooks himself up to a feeding tube. He's the smallest kid in his grade. His brother, a year older, is over a foot taller. I phoned the cousin. His voice sounded small – I could barely hear him. I spoke with his mother. I told her about the diet that had helped me. She'd heard of it. Chris's gastroenterologist said the diet wasn't good for his age, it didn't give Chris enough nutrition. Her gastro-enterologist was "renowned" for pediatric gastroenterology. Chris's mother was a registered nurse, she'd found the best doctor, she had inside knowledge. Her tone of voice told me to watch myself: she was a mother bear and I was stepping too close to the cub. I asked what kind of food Chris ate. She lightened up, told me he was able to eat anything he wanted. They wanted him to feel normal at school – not to have body image problems. I wanted to point out that eating anything during the day meant eating food which would not digest, that hindered any healing, that "normal" kids drank orangeade and ate French fries. I held my tongue. The "experts" had spoken, the mother's mind was made up. She would not consider alternatives.

Recently I've spent less time walking. Instead, I use the morning time to sit and write. Trying not to wake my wife, I go into the main room of our modest Brooklyn apartment. I set a laptop on a coffee table, kneel on a blanket, and write about my previous bad gut. I'm walking faster now. I want to get through this work day so I can return to the laptop. I haven't felt this frustrated since my years of being sick: when the doctor described my intestines as "bloody hamburger"; when I spent endless hours secluded away in my parents' basement, doubting I'd ever be able to live normally again. The following pages contain my experiences with ulcerative colitis. After I finish, I'll send the writing over to Chris and his mother. I cannot present them with studies. But I can present my experiences. I hope they help.

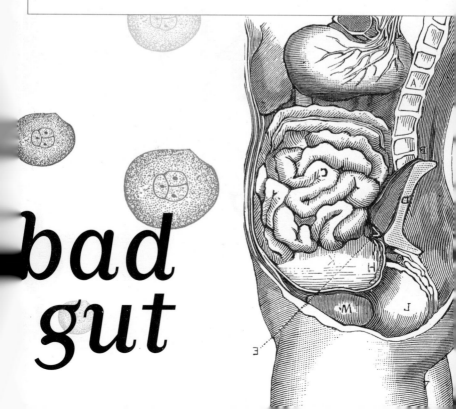

bad
gut

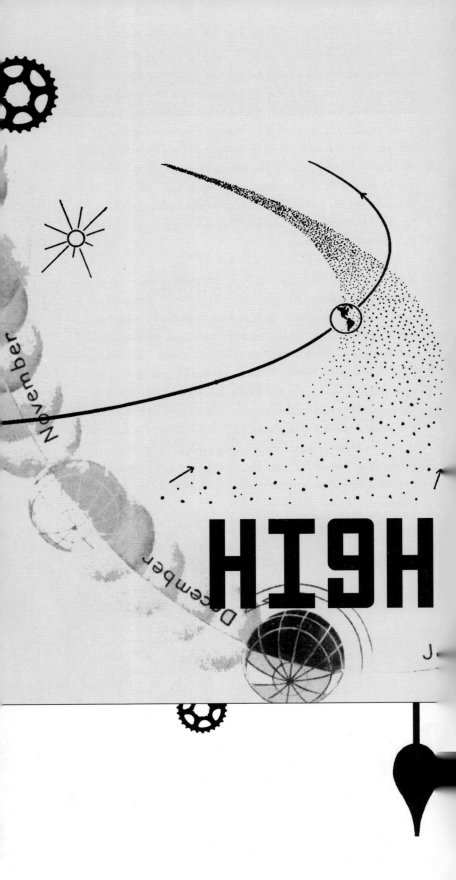

November

December

HIGH

J

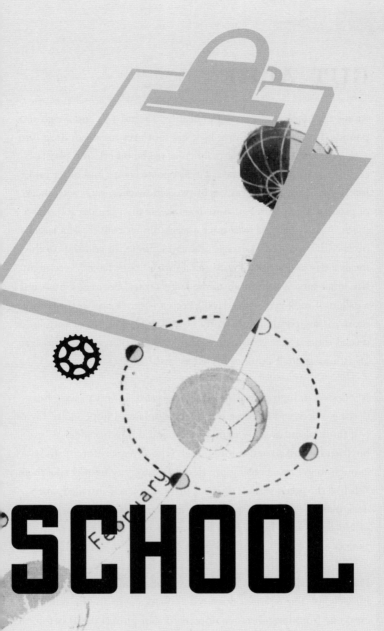

SCHOOL

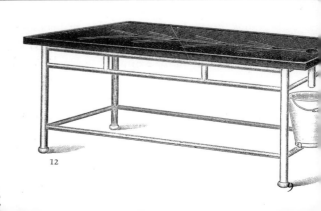

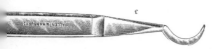

GUT ACHE

At age 17, I look upon myself as healthy. I stand 5'9" and weigh 160 pounds. I can do 17 pull-ups, kick my foot over my head, drop into a straddle split (one foot perpendicular to the other), and play soccer all day. I never drink soda; I avoid potato chips and other junk foods. My usual lunch consists of two sandwiches, each with slices of processed deli ham and American cheese on a grinder roll. For a snack, I eat apples. At least once a week dinner consists of a large pizza with pepperoni, sausage, and extra cheese. In addition to three meals a day and snacks, I consume bowls of corn flakes every night. My mom buys a half dozen of the largest cereal boxes at a time and a gallon of milk every two days. I keep a Kleenex box in the bedroom for my continuously stuffy nose. Taking a round of antibiotics several times a year is normal. I go for regular allergy shots and carry an asthma spray. I think of myself as healthy.

My desires in high school are straightforward. I want to have fun playing soccer and hanging out with classmates. I hope Jenny Taylor will think of me as more than a friend and dump her older boyfriend who'd passed through high school years before. I study enough to get by, choosing my classes because my friends take them. I dislike the green station wagon I drive, but a self-installed tape deck makes it OK. I fit somewhere in the middle of the social strata of North Haven High School in a mostly blue collar town of 23,000.

During the winter of my junior year, after school means going to lift weights. The assistant track coach owns a gym and he wants everyone from long-distance runners to shot putters to lift before the spring. After a day of English, math, history, anatomy/physiology, Latin and biology, we pile into one of our cars and head to the gym for 90 minute work-outs. This leads to the post-dinner feeding: two serving-size bowls of corn flakes each night covered with 2% milk. Except for the night before an anatomy test on the digestive track, I don't pay attention to the food after I eat. The body takes care of itself: in the morning I shower, go to the bathroom, and during the day I eat as much as I can.

For gym, I am a facilitator for the "Project Adventure" class. Instead of the usual activities of square dancing and dodge ball, this class involves rope courses, trust falls, and games which require the entire class to cooperatively solve problems, such as getting everyone over a 10 foot high wall.

During the previous year, the instructor showed us a movie about Outward Bound – a more intense version of Project Adventure. In the film a group of teenagers train to climb mountains and fly to South America to test their skills on a real peak. Although not survival programs, the Outward Bound courses put people through tough experiences so they gain mental hardiness. I find out that the Project Adventure class has money to help send people on Outward Bound courses. Thinking about how good I feel after gym class, I imagine that a trip would change my perspective on things. Sandwiched into a spring break at the end of March 1988, I sign up for a short canoe trip on the Rio Grande.

When I return from the trip I feel more relaxed, more alert. It has been my first time out of the suburbs – eight days of canoeing, camping, making every meal, struggling in the rain. Two weeks earlier I spent entire class periods looking out the window, watching an excavator and payloader digging a foundation. Before the trip I looked like everyone else in class, bored out of my mind and staring out the window. But now I'm laughing, happy to be indoors. For weeks I walk around with an idiotic grin on my face.

The Rio Grande trip has also brought along a case of stomach cramps and Montezuma's revenge. On April 12, 1989, the doctor prescribes donnatal, a pain-killer, for the cramping and loperamide for the diarrhea. Three days later, lab results come back and the doctor diagnoses a bacterial infection, shigella. One night on the trip I forgot safety precautions and swished my toothbrush in the waters of the Rio Grande. The shigella probably hopped on for the ride. I take a series of the antibiotic tetracycline. After that I don't seem to have any problems.

Two months after the canoe trip, in the beginning of June, I travel with a classmate to Washington, DC. Sponsored by the local Union Carbide plant, we spend a week with other high school students from around the country. The days are filled with workshops,

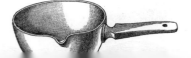

presentations by politicians, and lessons on how the government works. We sleep little (or not at all) and hang out in the dormitories all night. After arriving home, I receive another round of antibiotics for a respiratory infection.

For the summer, I work as an usher at the two-year old multiplex cinema. I make slightly less than my former stockboy/warehouse job at Xpect Discounts, trading off 10 hour days with one 15 minute lunch break for unlimited free movie tickets and a polyester suit.

I notice that if I drink orange juice first thing in the morning, my stomach begins to cramp, but otherwise I'm good. Every two weeks, I have popcorn duty at work. This means arriving in shorts and an old t-shirt, carrying a boom box, going to the windowless room upstairs and making enough popcorn to fill forty garbage bags. For quality control, I eat a handful of each batch. Once the bags are tied off, initialed, dated, and placed in storage, I go to lunch. Usually someone orders from a local deli and I have a sandwich waiting for me downstairs. Retiring to the back row of a show, I happily eat my meatball sub with Provolone cheese.

In September, school starts along with soccer. I love soccer. The year before I tore my quadricep early in the season, but now I play constantly. However, during the last few weeks, I have another case of Montezuma's revenge which, for the most part, I ignore.

After two more weeks pass, I notice blood in the stool. Scared, I go back to the doctor. Assuming that the blood is related to the post-Mexico sickness, he gives me an anti-diarrheal pill and a stronger anti-bacterial drug. I also take blood tests to check for other possibilities such as parasites. I accept the medicine, eager to continue with soccer.

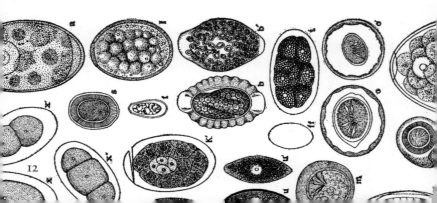

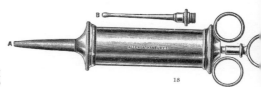

DIAGNOSIS

The blood and diarrhea continue for another week when the doctor calls to report that I tested positive for hepatitis. At his office, he explains that hepatitis causes fatigue and that rest provides the only cure.

According to the lab tests, I contracted the strain of hepatitis most often transmitted through sex or intravenous drug use. Due to the contagious nature of the disease, which can also be passed on through shared food, my family treats me as a leper. During meals my mom quarantines me at the counter while my sister, brother, and parents eat at the table. My dad warns me not to let anyone know about the disease, even my best friends.

"You'll see. I don't care how close they are. If they think you're really sick, they won't come near you. You also don't want the stigma of having a serious disease."

The hepatitis means no more soccer. I lie to the coach, telling him I have to sit out because of asthma. Driving home my body feels drained, hollow. For the next week I report to practice, sit on the sidelines with "asthma," and often leave early.

A close friend confronts me in the beginning of science class, angry that I've been sitting out of soccer practice. I told my other team-mates about the asthma but he doesn't believe it.

"You don't care at all, do you?! You don't care if we win or lose. You don't practice. People are losing faith in you."

Several classmates listen to this conversation. I want to defend myself and tell the truth about having hepatitis; but if my own family treats me as an outcast, I do not want to risk letting anyone else know. So I shrug it off.

The next week I again visit Community Care Plan (CCP), the local health maintenance organization, but I switch over to a different doctor. My father's co-workers tell him this new doctor is the best

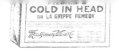

one there. The doctor questions my diagnosis.

"The blood test is positive for hepatitis but you don't have any of the symptoms."

He orders another blood test which returns negative. He concludes that the lab mixed up the first blood sample.

Not having hepatitis relieves me, but I continue to see blood in the toilet and the stomach pains sharpen. The new doctor, Dr. Klein, prescribes Rantidine, an anti-ulcer drug. Rantidine works as well as all the other medicines I have swallowed during the past weeks: it proves ineffective.

CCP becomes a second home. After school I navigate the green station wagon down the interstate to the Sargent Drive exit in New Haven. In the white-washed brick building I spend hour after hour in waiting rooms filled with the sick, lame, and wounded. I half-heartedly flip through months-old magazines. I should be tightening the laces on my cleats and running on the field, playing and joking around instead of sitting blank-faced, waiting. I sit and watch the dust float in the air, my mind turning numb. On my next visit the doctor prescribes antibiotics and tells me to avoid dairy products.

CCP is an early HMO, heralded because of the excellent doctors and the lower costs of having everything under one roof. In reality it's a combination of McDonald's and the Department of Motor Vehicles. Go to the desk. Announce yourself. The receptionist's fingers tap your name into the computer to confirm your appointment. Her practiced voice says, "The doctor will be right with you." *McDonald's.*

You sit for a few minutes. A few more. Pick through the magazines. Sit straight. Take a breath. Slouch back. Lean to one side. Prop up your head with your hand. Read a pamphlet. Check your watch. *DMV.*

A nurse calls you into the room. Thermometer in mouth. Blood pressure cuff on arm. Vitals noted. Symptoms listed. "The doctor will be right in." *McDonald's.*

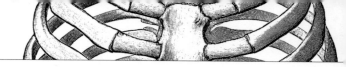

You sit on the fresh paper placed on the examining table. Boxed in a small square room. White tiles, white walls, white drop-ceiling with fireproof square panels. Look over at the boxes of gloves, the medicine bottles, the syringes. Everything made for easy cleaning and quick disposal. Look through another batch of months-old magazines, try the weighing scale again. *DMV.*

Door opens. Doc rushes into room. "How are you? Have the symptoms changed? What were your symptoms last time? Did the medication work? OK. I see. Here's another prescription. Have a good day." He checks his watch: well within his allotted six minutes. *McDonald's.*

I head to the front of the building, hand in my prescription order at Window 1, and go walking outside, killing time for the pharmacist to ready the order and announce my name at Window 3.

+   +   +   +

The school year marches on. It's SAT time. We line up with our sharpened pencils and photo IDs. Everyone's a bit nervous. I've been going through a book of practice tests. A woman talks about how much she drank last night – trying to make excuses. Someone tells the story of his brother's friend:

"He did acid the night before the test and blew it away."

"Sure he did."

"Well, he was smart anyway."

Most people stayed in to get a good night's sleep. I ate as little as possible for breakfast, but the gut pain stays the same way it has for weeks. I get through the test by concentration and dry swallowing half my daily supply of Kaopectate pills – the ones that I've been keeping in my pockets for weeks.

+   +   +   +

After a week on antibiotics, I come back to CCP feeling worse. Dr. Klein orders more blood tests and asks more questions before deciding to prescribe Metronidazole, or Flagyl.

"I'm going on a gut feeling that you still have something you caught during the Mexico trip. This drug is powerful but it should take care of any parasite or bacteria that still remains in your system."

He fills me with confidence that this will once and for all do away with the problem. He also prescribes Donnatal, a pain killer, to deal with cramping. With renewed faith in medicine, I thank him. I leave smiling, thinking I will feel healthy again. No more waiting rooms.

After two days of taking the Metronidazole, when I use the bath-room, the entire toilet bowl fills with blood. Keeled over from stomach pain, I go lie in bed and stare at the ceiling, afraid to move. If I eat, my stomach cramps and diarrhea immediately follows. I become afraid to eat. I lose so much blood...the entire bowl fills.

After another visit to CCP, Dr. Klein's schedules me for a sigmoi-doscopy, a procedure which involves sticking a tube into me with a camera to look at my intestines. I don't share thoughts of this madman's periscope with friends. I don't want the procedure but the alternative is continued bleeding.

During the sigmoidoscopy I keep my eyes closed and clench my fists tight enough to feel the blood flowing in my hands. I try to ignore what is happening, to put my mind somewhere else. After the doctor removes the scope, I open my eyes and see the nurse throwing out paper sheets covered with blood. It reminds me of the back room of a butcher shop.

I dress and go back to the regular examining room where my mother sits waiting. Soon the gastroenterologist, Dr. Montague, reputed to have graduated "top of her class" at an Ivy League school, enters. She had performed the procedure and with her hands washed, the diagnosis comes: "ulcerative colitis," a chronic disease with unknown origins that encompasses all of my symptoms.

In a rapid fire voice, she explains that I can never eat raw vege-tables, fruit, popcorn, or nuts again due to the severity of the intestinal damage. I face two choices of medication: "sulfasalazine or prednisone." Sulfasalazine, a milder drug has minor side effects,

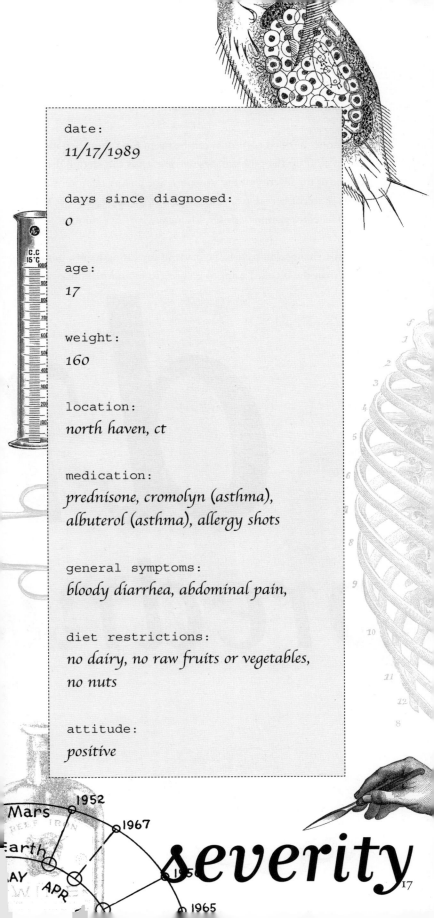

date:
11/17/1989

days since diagnosed:
0

age:
17

weight:
160

location:
north haven, ct

medication:
prednisone, cromolyn (asthma),
albuterol (asthma), allergy shots

general symptoms:
bloody diarrhea, abdominal pain,

diet restrictions:
no dairy, no raw fruits or vegetables,
no nuts

attitude:
positive

severity

the possibility of headaches and/or prolonging the problem. It would have to be taken for a long period of time. In addition, she mentions that it aggravates asthma.

Prednisone, purified cortisone, can be taken for a short period of time to clear up the problem. She recommends this steroid drug because of the severity of my situation. She doesn't mention side effects. I accept her advice, relieved that this whole episode is almost over. The conversation with Dr. Montague lasts five minutes.

A drastic change will have to be made in my eating habits, but it is better than the blood. I want to go back to my normal life.

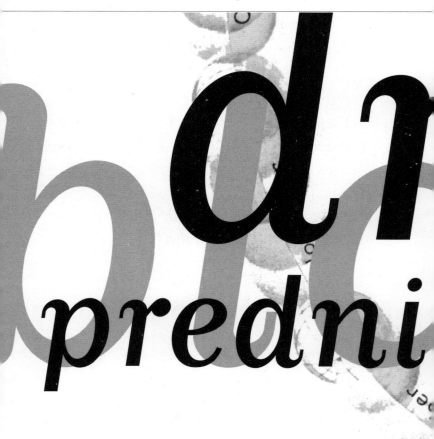

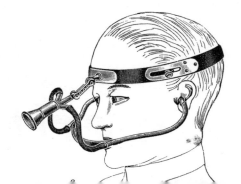

ituation

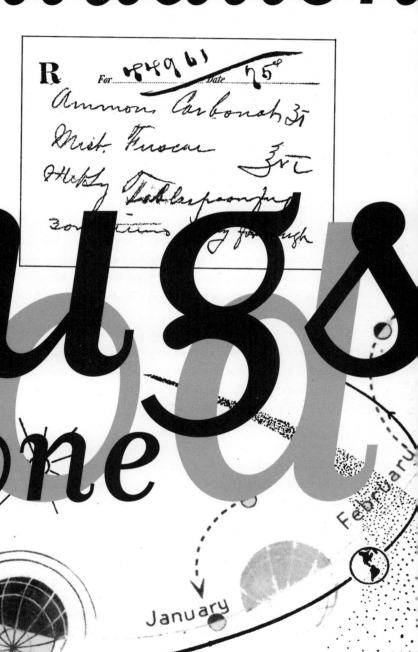

R For .... Date ....
Ammon. Carbonat 3i
Mist. Tusccu   3vi
M. ft. Tablespoonful
3om times a day for cough

ugs
one

January

February

TREATMENT

I start on 40 milligrams of prednisone. The normal human body produces 7 milligrams of cortisone each day to regulate metabolism. With nearly six times the normal amount of cortisone, my body acts like a record at high speed. My mind spins because of the drug, but my gut begins repairing.

The first night on prednisone I watch the movie *The Mask* on videotape. It tells the story of a boy with a huge, deformed face. Instead of sprawling on the couch or a chair, I find myself sitting on the back of the couch, or pacing around the room, or standing to cheer, cry, and sing. My sister stops watching halfway through, leaving the room to report that I've gone crazy. But I feel happy, the prednisone makes me feel as though I'm flying.

Within a few days, my stomach returns to normal. No more blood. No more running stomach. I return to school after missing a week and continue to take prednisone but at lower levels. Dr. Klein explains that the drug has to be tapered gradually.

"Since you are taking artificial cortisone, your adrenal glands stop creating it naturally. In order not to shock the body you have to decrease the prednisone dosage over a period of months, allowing the adrenals to 'warm up' to produce more cortisone. However, the gland won't restart immediately."

"A rule of thumb is that it takes as long to restart as the time you have taken the prednisone. So if you take prednisone for three months, eventually tapering the dosage down to zero, it will take the body approximately another three months to restart production. For those three months, with no natural cortisone being produced, the immune system will be weakened and you will be more susceptible to sickness."

During the bleeding and diarrhea I had been sedentary so I begin to lift weights. Being ill weakened me and I lift little more than half of the weight than I used the previous spring. But my muscles begin growing at a ridiculous pace. After a couple of weeks all my clothes

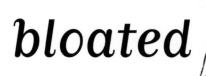

bloated

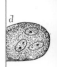

seem smaller. I measure my chest. It measures 45 inches when previously it had been 42. This comes with rapid weight gain, another cortisone side-effect. I don't like it, my body feels bloated.

+   +   +   +

In December, I start taking karate with Frank, a friend from high school. After abandoning soccer, I need to prove to myself that I can finish something.

The workouts at the studio are hard, I sweat as much as I did from playing a soccer game, and my muscles always feel sore the next morning. But after going, I become relaxed, happy. Although I'm far from my usual self, my health seems to be improving.

Around mid-December I have occasional stomach cramping but no other symptoms. One night, I run into a friend who was taking a break from college. The first thing he asks is, "Are you sick?"

"Why?"

"Your face looks swollen."

At home, I look in the mirror. My face has become a ball: round and double-chinned. My parents say they have seen the swelling during the past few weeks. It turns out to be facial mooning, a common symptom of prednisone use. It looks unnatural and increases my desire to get off the drug.

That night my father comes home disturbed. He has talked to a friend of his, a retired doctor. According to this doctor, people who remain on prednisone for over six months run the risk of having a shortened life span. I calculate I will be free of prednisone by late February, weeks before hitting six months. Yet the idea of a shortened life span stays in the back of my mind.

+   +   +   +

In the beginning of January, I come down with bronchitis. Dr. Klein gives me some penicillin. I'm now down to fifteen milligrams of prednisone.

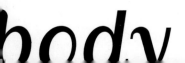

body

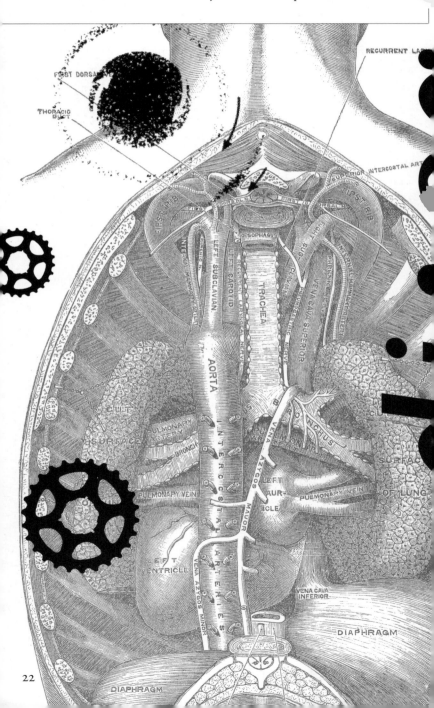

On February 10, 1990, I turn eighteen years old. My energy level has dropped and I'm not interested in celebrating my birthday when my family takes me to dinner that night to Captain Jimmy's, a seafood restaurant with dark wood and dim lighting. My grandmother comes with us so I try to act in an "up" mood.

When the waitress takes my order, I ask for tortellini. My mother interrupts, reprimanding me for ordering something with cheese. I'm still not supposed to eat dairy products.

I scan the menu. "I'll have the chicken."

Mom intervenes again. "You can't have that. Look, the sauce has cheese in it."

I shake my head as I re-read the menu. At first, I didn't mind the diet changes but it's become frustrating. Six months before I lived on pizza – with extra cheese.

+ + + +

During February vacation, I stay with five friends at a cottage situated next to the Vermont ski slopes. The second night there my head pounds and I'm the only non-drinker. (Can't drink with the meds.) After we all go to bed, I cannot not lie down without feeling nauseous. I climb down from the top bunk, go to the bathroom, and puke. I continue to do so every half hour. By the end I'm dry heaving. After each trip to the bathroom, I climb back onto the bunk bed and collapse, hoping my headache will go away. As the hours pass, I find it harder to climb back into the bed. Sometime, near dawn, I sleep. I don't ski the next day, watching TV instead.

+ + + +

The same week I go to Boston to visit my cousin at college. Walking through the train station, I become dizzy. Droplets of sweat trickle down my back, down my legs. When I sit down in the train I close my eyes to stop everything from spinning. I watch out the window as the train leaves New Haven station with its graffiti and dirt. I try sleeping but it doesn't work.

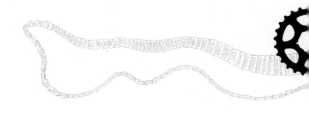

STILL SICK

After the week of skiing and visiting my cousin, I start going to the bathroom about six times a day. There is no blood and not as much diarrhea as in the fall, I just spend a lot of time in the bathroom. The prednisone dosage has tapered down to 10 mg a day.

I make an appointment with Dr. Montague, the gastroenterologist. She tells me that ulcerative colitis is a chronic disease.

"You are having a relapse. I'm going to raise the dosage of prednisone back to 40 milligrams. I'm also going to prescribe sulfasalazine. Once you stop the prednisone, you can continue indefinitely on the sulfa drug for maintenance."

In another appointment that week, Dr. Klein prescribes ergotamine, a migraine medicine, for my headaches.

I start getting spacey, even paranoid because of the increased prednisone. I fluctuate between hyperactive and lethargic. I can't go to karate any more. At school, I cannot see more than twenty feet down the hallway. Beyond that everything is blurred. I watch the ground to avoid losing my bearing and falling down. Sometimes I think people are getting ready to attack me. My "fight or flight" mechanism remains on high alert. Even with my body near collapse, my mind keeps spinning.

My stomach starts cramping to the point that I miss weeks of school. During the third week, my dad finds out through his secretary about a woman with ulcerative colitis who is now "cured." We call her up, me on one phone, my mom and dad on another. With my optimism already waning, the phone conversation destroys it. The woman says, "It was terrible and it took a long, long time to get rid of. I can't believe someone else has to go through it. I wouldn't wish it on my worst enemy. It took more than a year to go into remission and it can always come back."

She keeps repeating, "it was terrible... it was terrible."

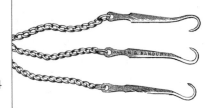

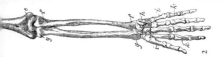

I'm eighteen. I'm supposed to graduate from high school in a few months. I don't have a year to waste.

After my parents thank her and hang up, they send me to pick up my younger sister from a friend's house. Getting into my parents' pick-up truck, I have a weird feeling come over me, a combination of anger, frustration, and prednisone. I drive recklessly, even after picking up my sister. I turn the radio to full volume, my sister starts crying out of fear, and I ignore her. After dropping her home, I skid out of the driveway leaving twenty foot marks.

I hit the highway and watch the luminescent green speedometer spin all the way around. I am going over one hundred miles an hour with tears streaming down my face. I cry so much the road blurs. Eventually I take my foot off the accelerator and rub my eyes with my shirt.

+ + + +

The next day I decide to help myself get better; I go to the town library and take out *Whole Body Healing*. It's a thick book which describes activities and treatments such as yoga, meditation, acupuncture and biofeedback. Most of it deals with healing the body with the mind.

These days I feel dizzy to the point of tipping over. With my veins flowing with prednisone, I decide to make another trip to the library. I start the truck and begin to slowly back up. CRUNCH!! The truck hits something solid but I see nothing in the rear view mirror. I get out and still don't notice anything. When I am two feet away, I see that I have hit my mother's car, the muffler of the truck breaking through the taillight. I did not see the car until I was almost touching it. What is wrong with me? I start swearing and kick the cinder block wall under the carport in vain. My mind is shot, why couldn't I see the car? I stop driving.

The next morning I ask my mother to drive me to the library of a local university so I can read more about ulcerative colitis. I discover that many blood tests I was given in the fall were useless because of medication the doctors had prescribed simultaneously. No tests for parasites or bacteria were valid because the medicine I was taking

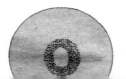

would mask the results. Most of the mistakes came from lack of communication between doctors. Also, I realize that not all doctors have knowledge of pharmaceutical effects.

Although not all the origins of ulcerative colitis are known, antibiotics, such as amoxicillin and penicillin, can trigger it. Before going to Mexico, I had taken penicillin for bronchitis. Dr. Klein also prescribed penicillin for me in January which could have aggravated the colitis. He should have consulted Dr. Montague: she was the specialist.

I read that prednisone's side-effects include dizziness, headaches, cramps, mood swings, high blood pressure, liver damage, a weakened immune system, osteoporosis, and many others.

+   +   +   +

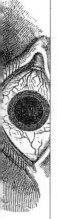

Whenever I can, I go out to the garage at night and hang up the punching bag I had bought the previous summer. I throw a side kick, followed by a backfist, then maybe a reverse punch, or elbow. Good solid combinations. Soon I lose any fluidity in my movements. I think about how unfair everything is and HIT! Think about the senior year activities I missed and HIT! Think about the hours I helped with the senior class play and now am dropping out of it and HIT! Think about the dozens of times nurses put the needle in my arm to draw blood for tests and HIT! Think about hepatitis and HIT! Think about how my accumulating absences might stop me from graduating and HIT! Think about how I missed my gold belt test in karate and HIT! Think about all the parties and times I was missing with my friends and HIT! and HIT! HIT! HIT! HIT! HIT! HIT! HIT! HIT!

By the time I go back into the house, I'm covered with sweat and I fall into bed.

+   +   +   +

For the next two weeks, my head pounds and I vomit for hours before it lets up. Stomach pain remains constant. Over the course of a day it changes from dull to intense pain which doubles me over. I can't do much. I'm too dizzy to read. The words blur.

hit hit hit hit
hit h.i.t

I'm run down and losing weight. One night I fail to hang the punching bag. I no longer have the strength to lift it. It doesn't matter; foam is falling out of my gloves; they are sparring gloves, not made for hitting the bag.

Dr. Klein removes anything at all from my diet which might aggravate the ulcerative colitis. He directs me to avoid meats and foods with corn syrup. With fruits, vegetables, and dairy products already gone, my diet consists of bread, water, and occasional soup broth.

+   +   +   +

The radio lessens the pain of the headaches or at least distracts me. But every time I turn it on, a slow song named "On the Road to Hell" plays.

Once in a while I think about college applications sent out last year. But they don't seem to mean much now. Pain makes everything fade away. Forget about college, I may have too many absences to finish high school this year. As far as I know it's the first time the vice president of the National Honor Society had to step in because of the president's failed health. At least I don't have to put on the bad tan suit again, for the induction ceremonies.

+   +   +   +

Each day, my goal is to get out of bed, take a shower, and get dressed. Sometimes it reaches late afternoon before I wake up. For the rest of the day, I either lie in bed or go downstairs and watch TV. For exercise, I stretch my legs by placing them on the rungs of a step ladder. In addition, I complete one hundred push-ups every other day.

No matter how many sets it takes, I always finish the hundred. Sometimes it takes eight sets, sometimes twenty. I cannot predict my strength. I shut my door, write 100 on the black board, turn on the radio, do as many push-ups as I can, chalk out how many I have left, wait sixty seconds, and start again until I finish. Sometimes I feel ready to pass out. But I always finish, no matter how long it takes. I feel that if I don't finish, I'll die.

hit *hit* *hit*

hit *hit*

It's 2 a.m. and it feels as though someone kicked me in the stomach. I begin wandering around my room and think about an afternoon conversation I had with my friend, Sam:

"How bad is it?" he asked.

"Mostly a lot of abdominal pain—"

"No, I mean, well – you're not gonna die, are you?"

"No, no, I'll be better soon."

"The other night Jim and I were talking. He said if you were gonna die, he'd help you for the rest of your life."

The subject changed fast, but it hits me now. I think about everything I'd do with a limited life. I'd call up Sam's girlfriend Sheryl in Utah and have her and her friend Julia fly down to escort Sam and James to the prom. I'd send Will to some Outward Bound program so he would be his old self and not as materialistic. Give Frank the punching bag. Make a will.

The hardest part would be trying to convince my parents that my dying wasn't that bad. When people die, it's hardest on the family. I would try not to suffer because I wouldn't want to see the pain on my mother's face. I would always try to be happy or appear to be. No problem. I could accept dying.

But while imagining this scenario, the ultimate pessimist in me comes out. What if I have a tumor or something and have to undergo treatment for a year or so. People would visit me, but the visits would become far and few between. All my friends would be in college. By the time I came back, I would be known as, "Oh, he was a nice kid. Too bad about the cancer." I'd have to reacquaint myself with everything and everyone. I'd rather die in a month than suffer for years trying to find my bearings. Dying and wiping the slate clean would be much easier. Less psychic pain.

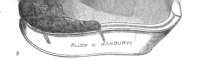

Visits to the doctor become more frequent. Dr. Montague breaks out of her rat-a-tat-tat speech pattern, nods sympathetically, and ups the prednisone to 60 mg – more than I took the previous fall. I still don't have diarrhea or blood, but I have bowel movements each time I eat and the stomach pain continues. I feel empty as if someone hit me in the gut with a two by four. Sometimes I cannot stand up straight or move without my stomach hurting. If I lie on the bed just right and take shallow breaths, I don't feel the pain.

Several times a week I have severe headaches followed by all night vomiting. After a while, I become too tired to get out of bed to throw up in the toilet. I line my wastebasket with a plastic bag and place it by the bed. Nothing makes the headaches go. I dissolve the blue ergotamine tablets under my tongue with no effect. My whole face tightens with pain. After vomiting for four to five hours, the pressure recedes and I fall asleep from exhaustion.

I look over the ulcerative colitis information again. With the amount of prednisone I am taking, my condition should have improved within two weeks. I am into week three.

Another trip to Dr. Klein provides hope. An X-ray of my intestines seems to show constipation and he suggests a laxative drink, magnesium citrate. He also gives me new information.

"Ulcerative colitis may alternate between constipation and diarrhea; your present condition looks to be the former."

This makes sense since my diet no longer contains roughage. Riding back from CCP, my mom at the wheel, I am overjoyed, finally – finally, a solution. I can go back to school, live a normal life, and get out of this zombie state. I go to sleep visualizing how great school will be next Monday. This is Friday night.

+   +   +   +

Saturday morning brings the worst pain in both my head and stomach. It won't let up. I cannot stay still and nothing alleviates it. After about an hour, my parents take me to CCP. Montague is on vacation but Dr. Harris, her partner, sees me.

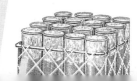

Harris orders more blood tests. This time I feel nothing when they stick the needle into my vein, the same spot punctured dozens of times in the last months. They see the pain in my face but cannot find the cause. They send me to the hospital emergency room. After three hours at CCP we spend another six in the waiting room of the hospital.

Never before has the pain been so bad. If I had the means, I think I would kill myself.

+   +   +   +

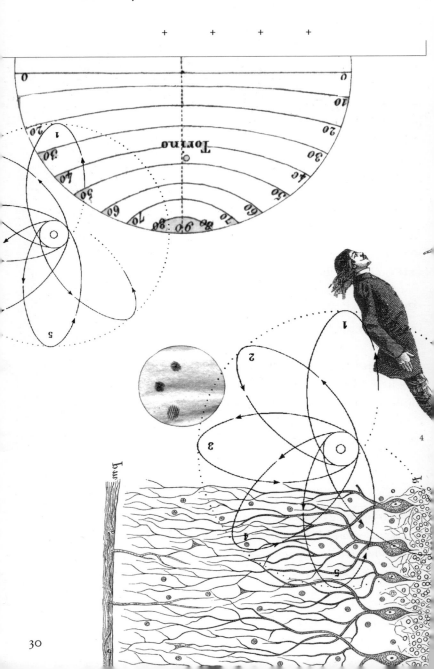

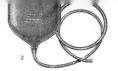

My blood pressure measures 160 over 110. The headache is now worse than the stomach pain. The place is overcrowded and I am put on a gurney in the hallway with most of the other patients. A nurse walks over and puts an IV in my arm.

I lie back in the bed while they roll me into an elevator and go up a floor. I get off the bed and they belt me into a diabolical looking table, including a strap across my forehead. A nurse comes over and says she's going to inject some kind of metallic substance into my veins. She warns that it may seem hot. I half-close my eyes.

The table I lie on slides back into a tube-like machine. From a booth in another room, the nurse tells me to stop breathing and the machine above me starts to whir. After a while, the blood in my veins boils. It's the hot you feel when you touch a steaming pan on a stove. When you touch a pan, you can take your hand away – but this is in my veins.

"Stop moving, we'll have to do that one over," says the nurse. I want to curse. My body wants to explode.

The test, a CAT scan of my brain, takes almost an hour and shows nothing out of the ordinary.

They wheel me downstairs, back to the center of the emergency room chaos, and draw blood for tests. They give me a spinal tap which involves sticking a four inch needle into one of my lower vertebrae and drawing fluid out to make sure I don't have menin- gitis. I lie in a semi-fetal position on my side as the doctor injects Novocaine to numb the area and lessen the pain of the big needle. Before he puts the needle in, to avoid the pain, I concentrate on flexing my leg muscles to the point they start shaking. I never feel the needle. He tells me that he stuck it in my back three times, missing the first two times, and not using Novocaine when he tried the third spot. The tests for meningitis come back negative.

Dr. Harris, Montague's partner from CCP, stops by the hospital and promises to find out what's going on with my body. He even questions the diagnosis of ulcerative colitis.

emergency

date:
3/17/1990

days since diagnosed:
120

age:
18

weight:
150

location:
north haven, ct

medication:
prednisone, sulfasalazine, ergotamine,
tylenol#3 with codeine, diphenoxylate

general symptoms:
abdominal pain; severe headaches;
unformed b.m.'s; blood in stool;
vomiting

diet restrictions:
no dairy, no raw fruits or
vegetables, no nuts, no products with
corn syrup, no meat

attitude:
exhausted, disoriented

MORE TESTS

With the pain lessening, we leave the hospital after 10 p.m. I hold a prescription for Tylenol with codeine to deal with any future headaches. In addition, Harris cut the prednisone dosage from 60mg to 35mg.

I go home feeling burnt out. I weigh myself and the needle stops at 150 pounds. My normal weight is 160. I haven't weighed that little in almost two years, since before going to the gym and eating all the extra bowls of cereal.

+   +   +   +

The hospital calls the next week to report a positive blood test. At last, I'll find out what's wrong. I return to the same emergency room. They put me in a room and tell me to lie down for a while. A nurse draws more blood to verify the test results. I wait with my mom for about two hours.

Harris stops by and talks. He theorizes I might have a stricture in my intestines which is causing the stomach pain. He goes on to say he knows I'm not a "malinger" because the doctor who gave me the spinal tap reported I have a very high pain tolerance. I'm annoyed: Who would fake something like this?

My mom goes to eat lunch and an intern comes by to take vitals. He asks what I plan to do in the future.

"Anything except medicine. After this, I don't want to spend any more time around sick people."

"You know, a lot of people decide to enter medicine after having a serious illness."

"Well, not me."

We continue to talk until the test results come back. Negative. The positive test was contaminated, probably by skin cells. Harris gives me a prescription for donnatal, a pain killer for my stomach, and schedules a series of tests.

+   +   +   +

Two days after the hospital I return to CCP for a GI (gastro-intes-tinal) series. After getting into a hospital gown, I drink a large cup of chalky liquid containing barium. The barium makes everything clear for the X-rays. Every fifteen minutes to half an hour the doctor X-rays my abdomen as the barium travels through my system. In between X-rays, I sit outside the door and glance through maga-zines. My head hurts again and I have tunnel vision.

In between one set of X-rays, the doctor lets me go outside and get some air. After putting on my sweatpants and my black pullover soccer jacket, I walk into the parking lot. The air smells of sewage from a nearby treatment plant. I look across the harbor to chimneys pouring clouds of fumes into the air. Litter dots the ground of the faded blacktop.

The tests, as usual, find nothing.

+   +   +   +

I cannot sleep, the medicine keeps my mind racing, I can't slow it down. At 3 a.m., after hours of mindless late night TV, I begin pacing around the house and find myself in the unlit living room practicing chon-gi, a karate exercise incorporating a series of blocks and punches while visualizing an invisible opponent.

For the next hour, I am in my own world of movement. For the first time I feel each motion. I perform each action with more fluidity and power than I thought I possessed. I fight the invisible opponent.

I return to my bedroom covered with sweat and worn out but my body still refuses to sleep. I sit down Indian style on the carpet with my back leaning against a closet door. Placing my hands on my knees, my palms facing the sky, I close my eyes. I let my muscles loosen. My head remains perfectly straight, aligned over my center of gravity. I have to know how to get better. I let my mind go, taking me out of the house, down the streets, past the town, into the sky, over fields, rivers, clouds, into the open. I see colors and faces, twisting and flying by, and when it all stops, I don't know where I am, but the answer lies before me. I don't see it, can't see it. It doesn't ease up on me, but comes all at once, filling my being, the answer is LOVE. I have to love everyone and everything. It all makes sense now. I stand up, renewed. The sun begins to peek through the window.

Anxious for my family to wake up so I can tell them the truth, I search for an activity to pass the time. I go outside. The backyard has been dug up and the topsoil needs raking before grass seed can be planted. Barefoot, my toes squishing in the soil, I fervently rake and rake and rake.

Returning inside, I decide to drive to get donuts for breakfast. This is my first time driving in over a month. The car moves much faster than I remember. Scenery flies by as I sit shaking and sweating. Inside the store, I feel as if everyone is looking at me, as if I have escaped from an asylum. I order a dozen donuts: black raspberry for my mom, honey dipped for my dad, creme-filled for my sister, and chocolate for my little brother.

When I return home, everyone is up. I talk at an insane pace, about staying up, and raking, and buying the donuts. Everything made sense before the reality of the day rushed back in. But I don't tell them about love. It doesn't make sense any more. I go into the bedroom and collapse.

+   +   +   +

The next day at CCP I have an ultrasound. The nurse rubs some sort of jelly on my stomach and passes an instrument over the jelly. Using sound waves, an image forms on the screen, a sonogram, of my insides. Nothing looks out of place.

For the next few days, the outdoor temperature rises and I spend time lying out on the carport roof, listening to the Walkman. I concentrate on relaxing my entire body and willing myself to get better.

Occasionally I open my eyes and look up at the sun. I visualize

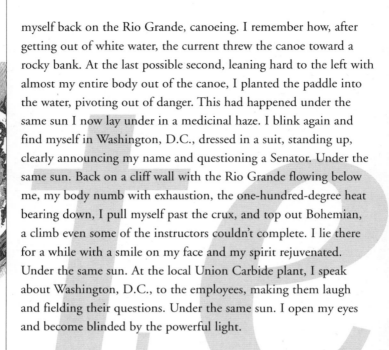

myself back on the Rio Grande, canoeing. I remember how, after getting out of white water, the current threw the canoe toward a rocky bank. At the last possible second, leaning hard to the left with almost my entire body out of the canoe, I planted the paddle into the water, pivoting out of danger. This had happened under the same sun I now lay under in a medicinal haze. I blink again and find myself in Washington, D.C., dressed in a suit, standing up, clearly announcing my name and questioning a Senator. Under the same sun. Back on a cliff wall with the Rio Grande flowing below me, my body numb with exhaustion, the one-hundred-degree heat bearing down, I pull myself past the crux, and top out Bohemian, a climb even some of the instructors couldn't complete. I lie there for a while with a smile on my face and my spirit rejuvenated. Under the same sun. At the local Union Carbide plant, I speak about Washington, D.C., to the employees, making them laugh and fielding their questions. Under the same sun. I open my eyes and become blinded by the powerful light.

What am I doing lying here? This isn't me. I shouldn't be passively letting the doctors run my life. They should have found out what was going on by now. I have to talk to Harris. I go inside and grab the phone. I want to be better. NOW. The phone clicks as the receptionist answers, Harris is out for the rest of the day.

+   +   +   +

The following week, I go for a CAT scan of my stomach. Before the test, the nurse gives me a drink which tastes similar to vodka and orange juice. Then I lie back and am strapped into the almighty CAT scanner. I am instructed to watch two lights above my head. One green, one red. I breath on green. After analyzing the results, a doctor calls to say nothing was found. It has turned into a regular procedure: take a test, find out nothing.

Harris doesn't find his stricture and becomes more confused. Though anyone can have ulcerative colitis, he says I don't fit the usual personality or ethnic type associated with the disease. My mother is part Swedish, part Italian and my father is Indian. No one else in the family has this type of problem.

Only one test remains, a colonoscopy which involves a six foot tube

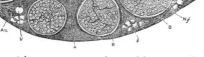

with a camera on the end being snaked through my intestines. Harris will look at my intestines through the camera and take tissue samples.

+   +   +   +

The drugs bloat my stomach. My waist has increased from 31 inches to 36 inches. At the same time, I begin to lose weight. I want to go back twelve months, right before Outward Bound. I was lifting weights for two hours every day and in the best shape of my life. Now I sit around with my bloated face and stomach, feeling like a freak. I have lost my body and, most of the time, my mind. What do I have left?

+   +   +   +

To prepare for the colonoscopy, in addition to not eating or drinking anything 24 hours before the test, I have to consume a gallon of Golytely, a powerful laxative, within a two hour period. I go downstairs to watch TV while drinking the dreaded gallon. After a while, I run to the bathroom every five minutes.

After the two hours pass I barely finish half the container. When I bring the glass to my lips, I start to gag. I drink regular water after the Golytely to get rid of the taste. My stomach starts cramping. I think about dumping the stuff into the sink but then I'd have to go through the whole process again.

Late into the night, I finish the Golytely. My stomach pain reaches a maximum. I head up to my bedroom, close the door, turn on the radio, and roll up into a fetal position on my bed. I feel only pain. I sing along with the radio, yelling the words to "Goodbye Ruby Tuesday" into the pillow, while tears stream down my face.

+   +   +   +

Colonoscopy day arrives. I put on the robe and lie down on the gurney. A nurse sticks the I.V. into my arm. She wheels me into another room where I am anesthetized.

I wake up back in the first room where my mother waits.

Dr. Harris, who performed the colonoscopy, enters. Unlike his usual demeanor, Harris speaks fast.

"The intestines look healthy with no signs of damage. He's ready to go back to school."

We start to ask questions but Harris turns to go.

"I have a busy schedule today."

Back home, I try to decipher the news. The stomach and head pain remain. My resting pulse still races at 120 beats per minute – during an anatomy lab last spring it was half that. According to all the books, if I had had a recurrence of ulcerative colitis during the past two months, my intestines could not be as healthy as the colonoscopy shows them to be.

Through another friend, my dad obtains the phone number of a gastroenterologist in Boston. I call her up and she says that ulcerative colitis cannot clear up so fast, that I couldn't have had a recurrence.

I fall sleep confused, a bit relieved, and determined to go to school the next day. My mother has contacted all of my teachers and the guidance counselor about my sickness. They are all understanding, the principal even makes an arrangement where I can come late to school or leave early, depending on how I feel.

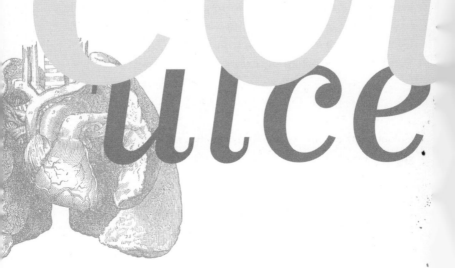

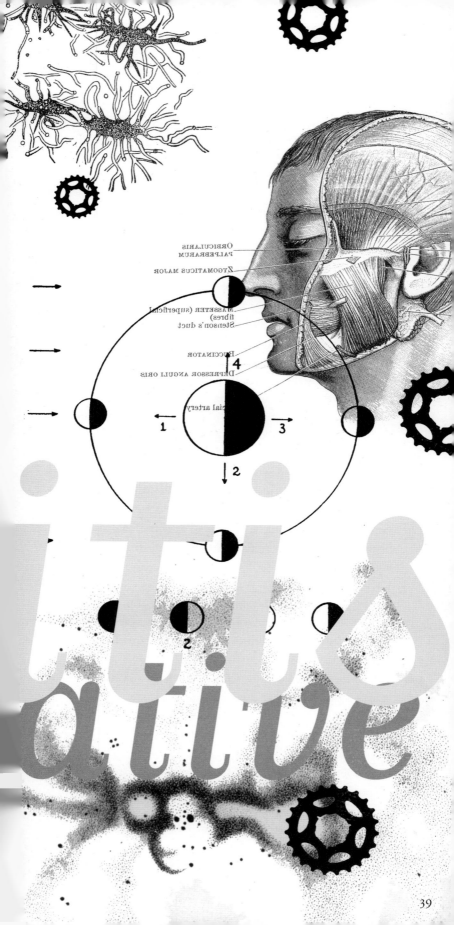

ORBICULARIS
PALPEBRARUM

ZYGOMATICUS MAJOR

MASSETER (superficial
fibres)
Stenson's duct

BUCCINATOR

DEPRESSOR ANGULI ORIS

facial artery

1

3

2

4

2

BACK TO SCHOOL

I wake up at midnight and cannot sleep because of stomach pain. Around 8 a.m., I eat breakfast, and after getting dressed, prepare myself to go to school. As usual, after I take the prednisone, I become wired and anxious: I have to slow down. I head to the garage, slip on the gloves which are temporarily repaired with duct tape, and start hitting the bag – which my dad helped me hang. Smooth combinations, one punch, then one-two, one-two-three, up to six. Each hit becomes stronger as I visualize going back to school. Fifteen minutes later, dripping in sweat, I stop and face the bag.

By the time I drive into the school parking lot, my third class, physics, has started. I wear a striped button down shirt with short sleeves. It was bought to wear to my grandmother's for Easter – to be put on during the car ride there and be taken off on the ride home. However, it's the only thing I am comfortable in. For months I've been sweating through layers of clothes: t-shirts and sweatshirts, t-shirts and sweaters, jackets. I can sweat through anything. Whether I am lying in bed or walking around, the sweat keeps coming. The button-down shirt seems baggy enough that it won't make contact with the soaked T-shirt beneath. My belly remains swollen out to 36 inches. With a pair of my father's size 36 pants, shirt untucked and hanging down, and a swollen, puffed-out face, I look into the window of the classroom for the first time in a month and a half.

As I turn the knob, my face breaks into a huge grin. Mr. Payne, the teacher, looks over and smiles. I enter, sarcastically apologizing for being late, and look at the class. Everyone starts clapping.

I spend the remainder of the school day talking non-stop. There are many people and teachers I haven't seen in a while.

+   +   +   +

For the remainder of the school year I receive special permission to come in late. I miss an average of one day per week going through withdrawal symptoms. Every third or fourth day I spend puking, dry heaving for five or six hours, shaking and sweating

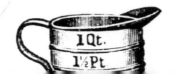

while coming off the meds which include prednisone, donnatal, and Tylenol #3 with codeine. After one dry heaving spell, as I lie exhausted in bed, with the curtains open and the sun coming in the window, I hear my mother crying.

Concerned, she had called Harris, telling him that I still wasn't doing well. He told her, "Your son's problem isn't in his stomach, it's in his head. I suggest you find another doctor." He then hung up.

Physically I'm a mess but I believe the doctor. I feel like a fool, a weakling. I become angry with my mom when she discusses my health. From that time on I become furious if anyone asks how I feel or how I am doing. The dizziness from the medicine and fatigue remains. My head spins around every day, my stomach remains distended, and my resting pulse never goes below 120. When I played soccer, my resting pulse was less than 60. A pulse of 120 is normal for someone running. With the medications, my body is running all the time.

At school I become a ghost-like presence, floating around, no longer involved with class, no longer part of any activities. Everyone has moved on. Summer is coming. Everyone is getting on just fine, looking healthy, knowing where they will be next year, and celebrating getting out of high school. Nearly everyone has suddenly outgrown it, they want to move on. That includes me, I don't want to go near the place.

+   +   +   +

Next week, after school, I have another appointment with Dr. Klein, the general practitioner. I skip the prednisone that morning so over 30 hours have passed without my taking the drug. Although I'm tired, my mind is clear, clearer than it has been in months.

My parents wait outside while I meet in the office with Dr. Klein. He suggests that I concentrate on tapering the prednisone and says it was good that the colonoscopy came out clear. I question him. During the past two months, I have had no symptoms of ulcerative colitis: Wasn't it possible that the prednisone could be responsible for the cramping and headaches? When the dosage was increased, I felt worse, and when it was increased further, I ended up spending a

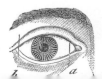

day in the hospital emergency room. The colonoscopy shows my intestines to be healthy, impossible if I did have ulcerative colitis during the past two months.

I earnestly ask him to tell me if prednisone could be the cause of the pain for the past months. He stays silent, immobile. I tell him I have to know for myself. He nods his head. He explains that ulcerative colitis is a "catch-all" term. People's symptoms of ulcerative colitis vary from mild to severe, with origins ranging from antibiotics to unknown. Doctors lump these problems under the name "ulcerative colitis."

I relate the news to my parents on the ride home. They note that Dr. Klein acted nervous while talking to them. He usually took more time to explain a situation. On this occasion, he spent about a minute with them and stumbled over a table leg while hurrying out the door.

Back home, I open the kitchen cabinet and start throwing out medication. I want to throw out the prednisone, but I cannot. Although prednisone caused problems, I have to taper off it or risk making myself worse.

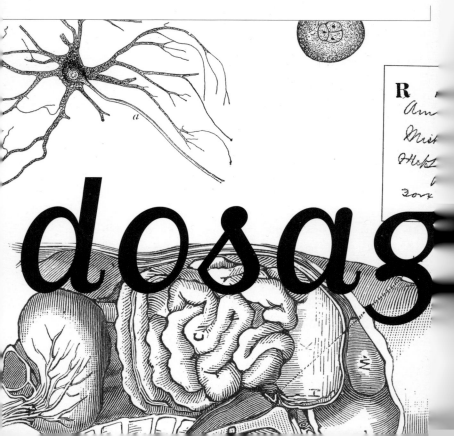

dosag

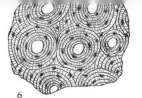

TAPERING

Each time I lower the dosage, I suffer withdrawal symptoms: headaches and vomiting throughout the night. When this happens I miss a day of school and use codeine to lessen the withdrawal effects.

+   +   +

Between Klein's and Harris's comments I remain unsure about what is going on – the lowering of the meds makes my head clearer but I am far from how I felt a year before. My parents help gather my medical records. Some of them we are not allowed access to but manage to obtain copies through a friend who works in the back office. Records of some appointments are missing, the ones where higher drug doses are prescribed. I type up a list of symptoms and medications.

+   +   +   +

In June, I make an appointment to see a more experienced doctor to review the records, one who has literally written the text books on gastroenterology. Flanked by a resident in training, this older doctor reminds me of Santa Claus. The patients before us leave thanking him; he acknowledges them with a kind eye. When our turn comes, we present him with the typed summary broken down by month. Each month, from March 1989 to June 1990, shows the diagnoses and prescriptions I was given. In addition, I give him copies of my medical files from CCP. After taking time to talk and ask questions, he says that initially, back in November, the doctor should not have prescribed prednisone.

Based on the initial sigmoidoscopy he says I should not have been given prednisone so quickly – that a milder drug may have worked. He suggests that it may be good to talk to some kind of counselor, and that he knows a woman who is good with teenage ulcerative colitis patients. I tell him it's not needed.

In a way, feeling vindicated, we leave with our sheaf of notes and papers. My father, after hearing about the doctor's opinion on the

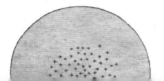

prednisone, looks surprised. From his experience working at a health insurance company, he says, "Doctors rarely speak against each other's work."

+ + + +

It's graduation day. Through a combination of forgiving teachers and long weekends of homework, I have mustered enough credits to finish. I'm lying in bed listening to Pink Floyd. I'm lying in bed while the sun streaks through the window.

Frank gives me a ride to the junior high school which is being used to group people for the walk out to the football field where ceremonies will be held. I sit with my home room, separated from school for months and suddenly re-appearing on the big day.

We're sandwiched into small chairs. The teacher is reading off the names, the alphabetical arrangement. We're walking down the hallway now. Homeroom after homeroom lines up. I'm dizzy, off-balance, but getting through. No one from my classes is around. Most people I know have last names closer to the front or to the back. There are faces I haven't seen in years. Lee walks two people ahead of me. Bobbling and shaking, throwing his arms out, teetering on one foot, then another. Wired, eyes crazed. We start moving again. While the bell rings, he tips back and kicks a hole into one of the windows lining the hallway. Laughing, he keeps moving, strutting ahead. No foot damage. Good boots – steel toed.

I keep walking, focusing on keeping my balance, getting out the door, getting to that chair. Sweating and stiff. No big day of relief or celebration here. I know my parents sit somewhere in the bleachers. My grandmother, my sister and brother.

On the stage, they're giving speeches, announcing names, the top ten going up, all the people from my classes. Everyone's cheering, everyone's going, getting their diplomas, their passes to get the hell out. Sitting. Focusing on keeping steady. I don't want to fall over when my turn comes. It's humid, sticky. Just take it slow. Yeah, that's it. Up the steps. Shake hands. Take the diploma. Exit. You made it.

44

+   +   +   +

It's mid-summer. There's a backyard party in town. Parents gone for the weekend. Keg in the shadows by a tree. The usual high school weekend. I'm talking to Ron. We were in the same classes through most of elementary school; during junior high and high school I didn't see him as much. In the seventh grade his dad died and he started hanging out in a fort in the woods by his house. It had electricity and plenty of beer. He seemed to lose his balance after his dad passed away but who was I to judge. My gut's still not right.

I talk to Ron about my last year. "I never know how I'm going to feel each day. I can't plan ahead. Some days I wake up and there's no energy or I'm puking all night. But the biggest thing is, I can't think ahead more than a day."

He shakes his head. "I couldn't live like that. I couldn't live like that."

+   +   +   +

I sleep a lot in the summer. No real job. I mow lawns, trim hedges, and do other minor landscaping at my parents' rental houses. I decide to go back to karate, I want to get my yellow belt. Six months have passed since I first went in the fall. I return in terrible shape, running out of breath fast, muscles knotted up. I begin stretching each day but can handle class only twice a week. The soreness lingers too long. Every few weeks, headaches and vomiting remind me that my body still has some adjusting to do.

+   +   +   +

I know it will take a long time to get back to normal. I have taken prednisone for nine months. It'll take up to another nine months before my body will produce cortisone naturally.

When I stand on the scale, the dial hits 145 pounds. Along with my losing fifteen pounds, my strength levels remain low. I have stretch marks on my chest and legs from the previous winter when my body ballooned with prednisone use.

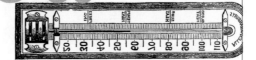

+   +   +   +

In July I am nearly drug free, down to 5 milligrams of prednisone.
While tapering off the drug I see a new gastroenterologist,
Dr. Brennan. He listens for a long time during the first appointment. When he finds out my low dosage of prednisone, he tells me
to stop the drug completely. However, he finds blood in a fecal
smear, re-starts the sulfasalazine, and schedules a sigmoidoscopy.
In addition, he prescribes Rowasa enemas. The tissue samples from
the sigmoidoscopy show "severe, acute and chronic inflammation"
indicative of inflammatory bowel disease. Tests for parasites find
nothing. Brennan, eyes fixed and serious, tells me what to expect.

"It's a lifelong disease. You can minimize flare-ups by keeping up the
medication. But this isn't going away."

"Thank you." I'm polite and upbeat, because I know it's a mistake.
I deny to myself that I have this disease. It has to be a milk allergy
or something else the doctors are missing. Once they find it, all of
this will drop away.

I think of a cartoon where Bugs Bunny is hurdling off a cliff in an
elevator toward certain death. But at the last moment, Bugs opens
the door and calmly steps out as the elevator crashes to the ground
behind him. I have dreams of recovering fully, stepping away from
this disease, leaving it behind.

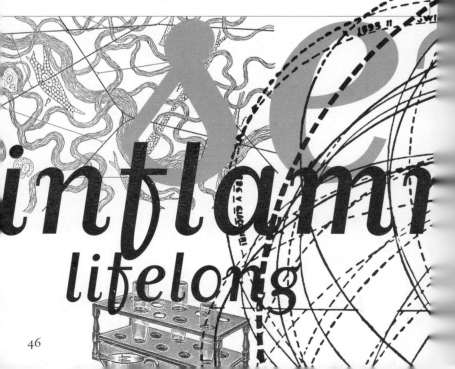

inflam

lifelong

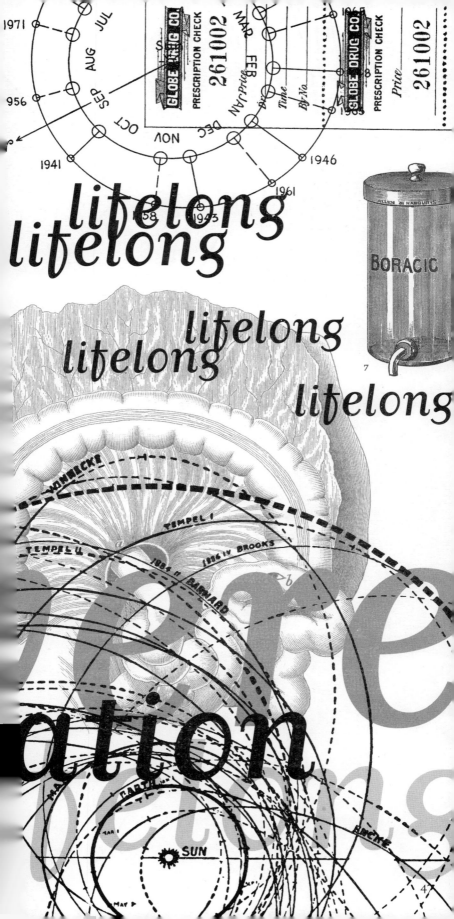

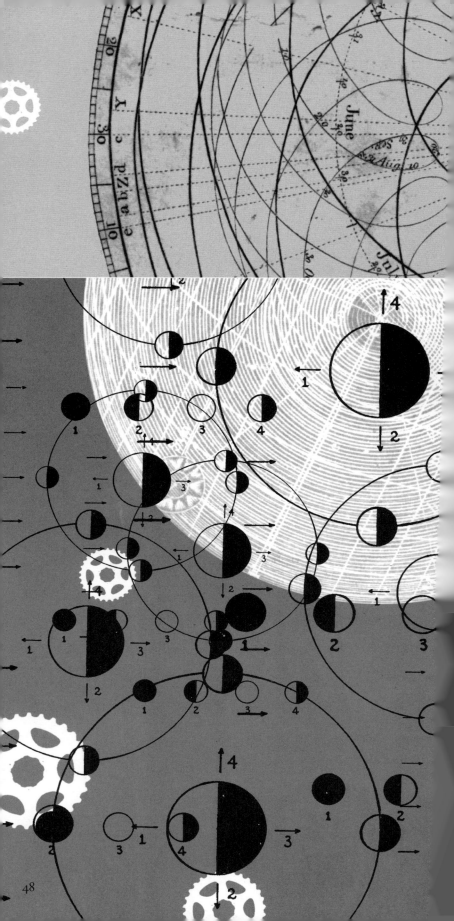

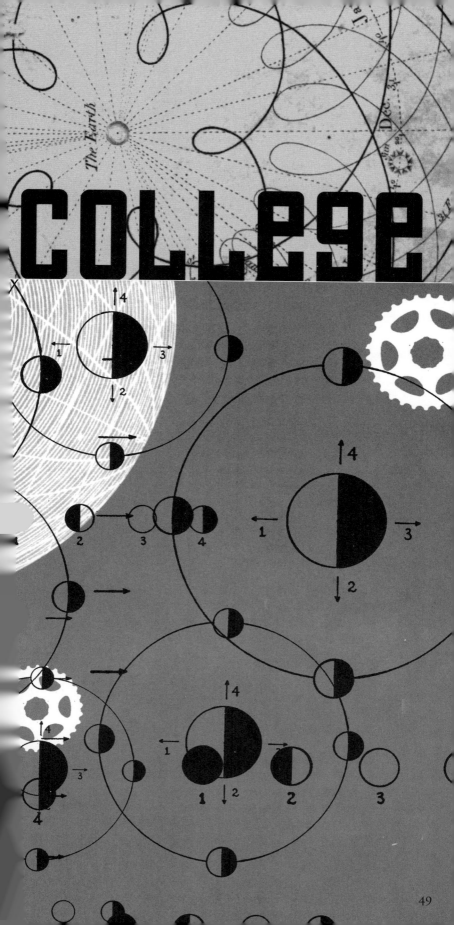

COLLEGE

STARTING COLLEGE

When I leave for college I take summer clothes, winter clothes,
a portable stereo with a dual tape deck, a six-foot step ladder for
stretching, and, hidden in a triple layered plastic bag, I bring
four boxes of Rowasa enemas. In my single room I place them in
the back of an overhead storage cabinet, accessible only via the
step ladder.

The first night brings the sound of bagpipes as a frat comes by with
its traditional "mobile keg" traveling on a supermarket shopping
cart. In our hallway we paint the walls, play soccer, discuss sex,
politics, and go to party after party – always laughing. As a community service project for a class I attend an AIDS dance-a-thon in
New York City accompanied by five women. Classes are tough but
English is my favorite – the teacher incredible. My Critical Issues
seminar makes me question my entire view of society and self.
Every Tuesday night after class I sit in my room for an hour,
piecing it all back together again, struggling, expanding, coming
out wiser, stronger. The cafeteria food doesn't agree with me, but
I make friends with the owner of a local deli and secure a daily
supply of meatball grinders – minus the provolone cheese.

I don't talk about being sick the previous year. I'm trying to put
it behind me. I am public about avoiding milk, saying I have an
allergy. Someone else on the hallway has a lactose intolerance
problem. At a pizza party, he watches me swallow Lactaid pills
with each slice, trying in vain to digest the cheese.

I don't try the pizza again, but day to day I cannot depend on my
energy. One day we play soccer and I feel good – untouchable.
On other days I feel foggy, clumsy, not able to wake up.

+   +   +   +

You squirt the Rowasa before going to sleep, and attempt to hold it
in through the night. In the morning it squirts out again: thick
brown liquid that stinks. Despite the Azulfidine and avoiding dairy,
my stomach feels full or bloated most of the time.

The energy of the people on the hall keeps me going. Without them, if I lived back home, I might have faded out, faded away, but here there's always something new.

+   +   +   +

After the summer, and getting off the prednisone, I sleep all the time. My adrenal glands have yet to "warm up." The college schedule lets me nap between classes.

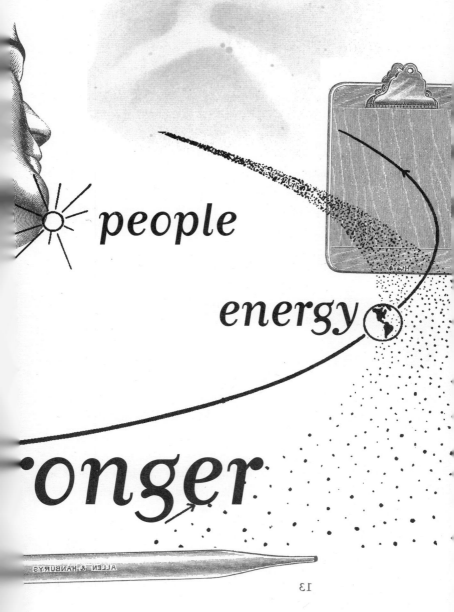

people

energy

onger

12

NEW MEDS

In October, my gastroenterologist, Dr. Brennan, stops the Azulfidine and introduces me to Pentasa. Within days, my stomach becomes unsettled. Diarrhea becomes the norm. I begin heading toward the dorm's basement bathroom more often, not wanting to use the same place six times a day. I try to ignore it, I never look down, I don't want to see the blood in the bowl.

I question Dr. Brennan about whether Pentasa might be partly responsible.

"I don't know how it can make you worse. It only contains the active ingredients of Azulfidine."

I feel foolish and keep taking it. I ignore my health. I want to spend time with new friends, hear stories, move on with my life.

My strength fades. I go to lift weights in the school's new gym and find myself much weaker than in the summer. After taking a shower and changing, I walk outside and become dizzy. I half fall onto a bench, blacking out for thirty seconds. Despite telling myself I'm OK, my body isn't buying it.

+   +   +   +

During Thanksgiving my father informs me that I will be going to a different school for the spring semester – one more well-known where I'd been accepted off the waiting list as a January freshman. Before starting in the fall, I planned on attending the other school. But within weeks I had decided to stay where I am – a decision strengthened by my mid-semester visit to upstate New York and the place I was accepted for January admission. I have made new friends. I want to hang out with Dave Mulé a few doors down, with Sid across the hallway, with Joe Suh who started the Tae Kwon Do club. I go with him to get funding. We have a high kick contest on the hallway. From stretching with the ladder, I can touch the exit sign hanging from the ceiling with my foot.

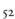

My protests to my father fail. I seek other avenues. I meet with the Dean to see about loans and financial aid. She sympathizes, but I would have to become an independent resident and show tax returns to apply for aid. That means taking at least a year off. I try my father again, armed with statistics of people applying to grad schools, college ratings, studies of how small class size is a positive thing. Logic fails. He tells me how he once heard of the bigger university while in India, and now finds it amazing that a son of his – he, a man from a dirt village – might attend that school. I try to find ways to get tuition money for the following semester. The most lucrative plot involves the entire hallway donating to a sperm bank. Nearly everyone signs on – it's a good cause, but only a few weeks remain in the semester and the donations will take several months.

With the anger and frustration, my gut worsens. I find out that a friend of my aunt who has ulcerative colitis became worse on Pentasa. After hearing this, I switch back to Azulfidine which helps. The Pentasa was no good. During break I spend much of the time hitting the punching bag. While eating, my fingers shake – nerves frayed, damaged from hours of punching.

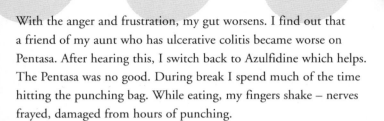

protests

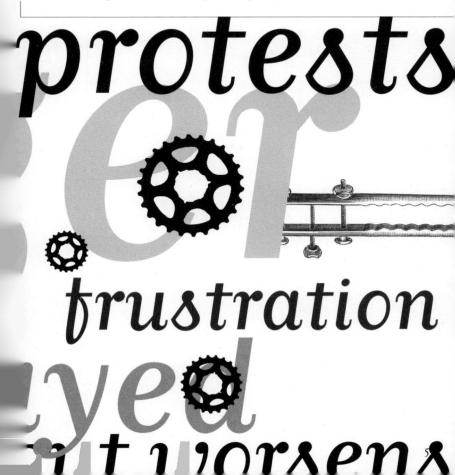

frustration

yed

ut worsens

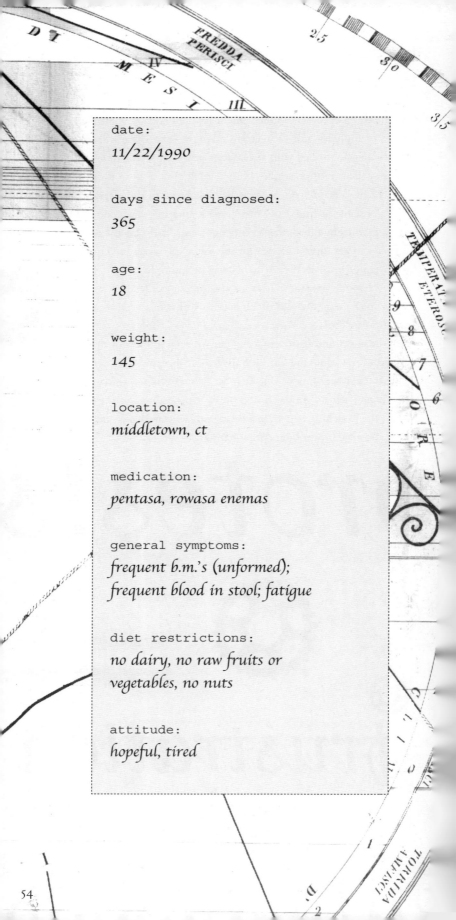

date:
11/22/1990

days since diagnosed:
365

age:
18

weight:
145

location:
middletown, ct

medication:
pentasa, rowasa enemas

general symptoms:
frequent b.m.'s (unformed);
frequent blood in stool; fatigue

diet restrictions:
no dairy, no raw fruits or
vegetables, no nuts

attitude:
hopeful, tired

NEW SCHOOL

The new school starts out cold. I wear a wool hat to go outside.
The dorm is at the outer edge of campus and divided into "suites"
instead of hallways – architecture conceived after the late 1960s to
stop large meetings. Groups within the suite have formed during
the previous semester and most people seem OK. I'm able to get
a single room to accommodate my triple-wrapped boxes of Rowasa.
I take a large sketching pad and marker which hung outside my
door during the previous semester and place it on my new door.

The first night, as I lie in bed exhausted, someone stands outside
reading the pad, "Welcome, RAY–MIN! I'll welcome RAY-MIN!!
Listen to this name! I'll welcome him! How's that for a welcome!
Maybe I should welcome him some more! I'll piss on his door!"
I get up and begin opening the door. Someone runs to one of
the other three rooms in the suite, a door slamming behind him.
There was no time to piss, but a bagel with cream cheese has
been smeared on the pad. I walk over to the door that had been
slammed and knock. I know Bill and Jon live here although they
haven't been seen yet this semester since they are pledging a frat.
Bill agrees to clean the cream cheese, and says it was a joke. I rip
off the page and throw it into the trash. When Bill's door closes,
he laughs hysterically.

I pass the first month fatigued, with anger simmering beneath the
surface. The long walks to class exhaust me and I lose more weight.
But the food is amazing and in February I feel energy start to return.
Perhaps my adrenals have started to normalize.

My stomach still feels heavy, eating always leads to gas and bloating.
I keep to a strict diet of no dairy, no fruit, no raw vegetables, and
no junk food. At least 75 percent of my food intake consists of
complex carbohydrates – bread, pasta, and occasional cereal (in a
bowl of orange juice). Squirting in the Rowasa continues through
February. The worst part about it is the morning. Expelling the
liquid is loud – and it stinks. In elementary school having this
kind of gas could make you a hero but now it means something
has gone seriously wrong.

SKINNY LEGS

When the spring sun first peaks out, I find a secluded spot on
the back landing of a small observatory. If it's warm enough, I lie
down and stare at the sky for hours, trying to make sense of the
past two years.

In my section of campus, a faculty member visits each of the dorms
once a week to chat with students about anything at all. Not many
people come to these things but a woman in the adjacent suite drags
me to a meeting. The faculty member, a woman in her early 40s,
entertains everyone with funny stories and takes an interest in all
of our activities. I go a few more times and when the temperature
warms up, I arrive there wearing shorts. In the middle of a conversation, a woman in the room lets out a loud yelp. Everyone turns
toward her.

"Oh my God!" She covers her mouth with her hands.

The faculty member asks what's the matter.

"Look at his legs!" She points towards me and all eyes turn.

"They're so skinny! Are you sick?! You look like you're starving!"

I don't know what to say. I shrug and the moment passes. Later
that day I look in the mirror. My legs have always been skinny
due to my dad's Indian genes but now I have no calves, just a vein
where the muscles used to be. The cross-campus walking has worn
them down to nothing and for the rest of the semester I become
overly self-conscious. I begin working out at the only free gym
on campus, using the one piece of equipment, an old universal
machine, to strengthen my legs. I also play in some pick-up soccer
games. The calves don't improve much but the situation seems to.

+   +   +   +

My father relents, saying that if I finish the semester and want to
go back to the other school, it's my choice. I decide to go back.

The housing lottery has started at both schools and I pass up getting together with people in my current dorm to move back with people from the old hallway. I cannot wait to leave. Early incident aside, the big name school lacks the energy of the smaller one, both in the classroom and out. There isn't the same impetus to question your own motivations and values.

On the day of the big school's housing lottery, I speak with my mom about the next academic year, telling her whom I plan to live with when I return to the first school. Her voice softens. "Didn't you father tell you? You're not going back."

"That's not true. I spoke to him last week. He gave me the choice."

"But he assumed you'd make the right choice."

I hang up the phone, look at the clock and curse. Only a few minutes remain in the housing lottery. I jog towards the building, jumping in the air and slamming a parking sign with the edge of my hand along the way, leaving it rattling. Few housing choices are left. Rooms remain only in the biggest dorm on campus. From the map of the building I choose a room on a dead end basement hallway, situated between a small gym and the cafeteria. I don't believe I'll ever have to live in it. But if I do, I decide to isolate myself, to concentrate on studying and keeping healthy.

I'm no longer taking the Rowasa but keeping on a steady dose of Azulfidine. The bowels still don't work well, I have lots of bloating after nearly every meal, and, after eighteen months, still no solid bowel movements.

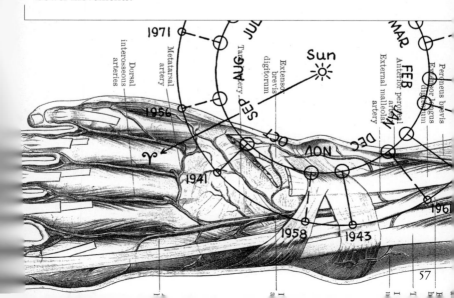

WAREHOUSE

When the semester ends I head home, ready to re-start my life.
My attitude toward ulcerative colitis convolutes over time. In high
school, armed with a vocabulary from classes in biology, chemistry,
and anatomy & physiology, I used a college library to dig up as
many articles as I could on colitis. I hoped to find a drug treatment,
diet regimen, exercise program, or other method to treat the
condition. These scientific papers re-iterate the lack of a cure, the
chronic nature of the disease, and the high chance of colon cancer.
Since they provide no comfort, I pretend they don't exist. I ignore
Brennan's speech about the chronic nature of the disease and
instead cling to Harris's words that the disease is all in my head.
I think that if I reduce my stress, the ulcerative colitis will go away.
It's up to me. I read in several places that exercise is one of the best
methods to relieve stress. In addition, the last time we met, Dr.
Klein said I might never return to my former level of health. I want
to prove him wrong.

For a summer job, I work at the warehouse of an electrical contractor whom my family knows. Jobs are scarce this summer and this
one pays a kingly $8.50 an hour. On my first day, Sal, the wiry, 57-
year old warehouse manager tells me to hop into a battered Ford
pick-up truck, and we head to a supplier. He introduces himself
with a scowl, "So you go to college. I've had college kids before..."
My fresh-out-of-the-box work boots don't help the situation.

After picking up some parts, Sal takes me on a walking tour of
the warehouses. The final one, big enough to have a horizon line,
contains the "remains" of several big jobs: piles of tangled wire
and scrap wood; work lights temporarily mounted on hastily nailed
together stands; battered, dented large tool boxes for locking up
equipment on site; and all manner of debris. As a first assignment
Al tells me to clean it up. The boots dirty up as I salvage wires,
disassemble lights and rebuild them with proper stands, scrape
and repaint the boxes, organize, and sweep the whole place. After
the first week the routine becomes steady: preparing deliveries
for sites, receiving orders and taking them into the warehouse with
the forklift, going to the sites, moving pipes and boxes, and doing
smaller-scale clean up jobs similar to those of the first day.

My gut seems OK. There's some discomfort, but as long as I keep moving, it doesn't bother me. There are still no solid bowel movements but I'm used to that now.

In addition to working at the warehouse, I begin lifting weights with Frank, a friend from high school. We follow a strict schedule of lifting three days in a row and then taking a day off. From another friend we borrow a squat rack and put it into my basement. Of the three day cycle, the first exercise on the first day is the toughest: clean and press. This means lifting the weight from the ground to shoulder level and then pressing it straight overhead. After that we complete upright rows, lateral raises, two biceps exercises, and two triceps exercises. We do five sets of everything. During the first weeks of lifting, my arms tremble while moving boxes in the warehouse.

After work at the warehouse, I have to push to do the lifting but I want to blow away all feelings from the previous year and start over, regain my health. One night I come home from the warehouse and fall asleep sprawled out on the kitchen floor. I miss dinner but when Frank arrives an hour later I still complete the work out (and eat a late meal).

Sal treats me well and I work hard to keep up with his tremendous energy. Occasionally he gives me a good job, such as bringing the boss's daughter's Porsche to the shop. On another day, we deliver fixtures and mattresses to the boss's son's house which is still under construction. Overlooking the ocean, with two story high panels of windows, the house appears ridiculously big for three people. I can't see to the end of the hallway and there's a room for a child's carousel. As Sal looks at the ocean, he remarks, "Kid, you and I will never see this kind of money..." The boss's house is next door. Of similar size, it has the profile of a ship.

My lunch, similar to my high school lunches, consists of two subs with salami or ham – but no cheese. My stomach feels bloated but I start looking into the bowl again. Usually, I have only gas and mucous. A few times blood – but this only makes me lift harder – and angrier.

weights

I go away on a couple of weekends. Once to visit some first semester college friends having a party. Another time I drive to a music festival in Vermont. Both times I realize the frequency that I use the loo, especially in the morning. But I assume the problem will resolve as I kept lifting – it has to. By the end of the summer I weigh nearly 160 again and receive a positive sendoff from Sal.

"Kid, I hate to see you go. If you could stay, I would train you as an apprentice."

I thank him and head back to school.

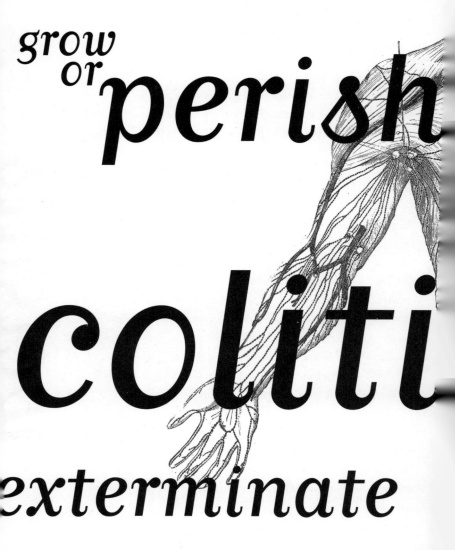

grow or perish

coliti

exterminate

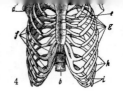

WEIGHTS

The remainder of my college career has a singular underlying focus which results in seemingly inconsistent behavior. I want to emulate a cowboy in a movie. I don't want to know how to ride. I don't want to hold myself like Clint Eastwood or shoot like the Sundance Kid. I want to emulate Curly in the film *City Slickers*. Jack Palance plays Curly, a leathery old cowboy who works in the 1990s by taking tourists on cattle drives. At one point in the film, Billy Crystal, playing a confused New Yorker, starts making fun of Curly not knowing that he is within listening range. When Billy Crystal realizes his mistake, he shakes with fear, waiting for Curly to kill him. Instead, Curly says: "I shit bigger than you" and rides away. That's what I want to do: shit big, huge! I'd be happy with a few days of solid BM's (bowel movements).

Working in the warehouse during the summer has made me stronger, perhaps stronger than before the illness, but it hasn't cured me. I continue with the stress theory. Stress causes the disease. Exercise reduces stress. Therefore, more exercise will eliminate stress, causing the disease to disappear. In the spring semester of my sophomore year, I want to get strong enough so that all sickness leaves my body and my digestion normalizes. If there are any residual emotional effects of colitis, I plan to blast through them, emptying myself of doubts. I sign up at the gym in my dorm: "Fitness North." It contains an old universal machine, a newly repainted squat rack, and other hand-me-downs from the varsity gym, a place as expensive as a private gym and almost as far. Varsity gym is at least a 45-minute walk, up and down, over the gorges, through the snow, only to wait in line at each piece of equipment, behind the football team, then the soccer team. Instead I use Fitness North, this hole in the wall in the back corner of the dorm which was once part of the post office. With a modest usage fee, cheap carpeting, fresh paint on uneven walls, a gym sock smell, old equipment, and a loud stereo complete with tape player, it's the perfect place to exterminate colitis.

I train with Dylan who's part of the group I hang out with in the dorm. Forgetting about any previous lifting experience, we put our trust into a small booklet outlining an 8-week program. The exercises guarantee that our muscles will either grow or perish.

The booklet calls for performing at least four sets in a row without stopping. The first cycle of chest exercises starts with dumbbell flyes. I take a dumbbell in each hand and lie flat on the bench so I'm staring at the ceiling tiles. Then it starts: hold the weights overhead with arms nearly straight and palms facing each other. I open my arms out as if I'm going to hug a redwood and then bring the weight back overhead again. After six reps, when the weight become too heavy, Dylan spots, assisting me in getting a couple of easy extra reps. He continues to spot until he's lifting almost all of the weight. I stop only when I can no longer lower the weight safely. By then sweats starts showing on my face, my arms shake, and I switch to a lighter pair of dumbbells. The process repeats itself. After putting the dumbbells down I slide back on the bench and immediately start bench pressing a bar which we've already prepared. Again, the weight starts heavy, then half is stripped off, and then half again – only the bar. By the end I'm sweating hard and need to catch my breath. For all five sets, the two dumbbell flyes, and three bench presses, we go to failure on both the lifting and lowering. We take turns, the spotter working almost as much as the lifter. In the booklet, those five sets are considered one "cycle." We complete four to six "cycles" for each muscle.

For 2 to 2 ½ hours a day, six days a week, we focus on the routines. The only distraction comes from flipping over the "rocket" tape, a cassette kept near the stereo which feeds a steady stream of Guns-n-Roses, Public Enemy, and anything else loud and fast to keep our thoughts away, to keep the adrenaline going strong.

We eat dinner at 4:30 p.m. each day, at the opening of the dining hall doors. We head to the gym around 6 p.m., when there aren't many people so we can set up all the extra bars and dumbbells needed for continuously cutting the weight in half.

We eat 4,500 calories a day, 75%-85% carbohydrates (mostly complex), 10%-15% protein, and very little fat. According to a friend who's taking a sports nutrition class and analyzes our diet on the computer, this makes a good combination – a good athletic diet. I skip classes in order to sleep before going to eat and lift.

75lb.

80lb.

Each night I cook a pound of pasta – half for me, the rest shared by people in the hallway. My body loses any remaining fat and veins start coming out of my chest. We increase flies from 30 pound to 70 pound dumbbells. The weight stack on the lat machine becomes too light and we add plates on top. My skinny legs squat 300 ten times and Dylan does 500 two times. Shoulder shrugs go over the 300 pound level and sit-ups on the incline board are done holding 45-pound plates. At the end of the program, I am two pounds above my high school weight of 160 but am far stronger. Dylan makes similar gains. We congratulate ourselves and continue going to the gym but at a sustainable rate: four days a week for 90 minutes.

With the 4,500 calories – extra pasta, early dinners, and a honey bear emptied each day to flavor bread – my body takes in more energy and breaks down more food because it has to. However, despite sweating out all emotion, breaking through personal pain barriers each workout, and not doubting for a minute that I can complete the program, my digestion does not improve. At the end I am no closer to being Curly in the movies. My bowel movements remain unformed, perhaps even worse than before.

During the day, the building staff opens a service door on my dead-end basement hallway. The door accesses a passage connected to the section of the building housing the post office. It also contains an unknown loo – an extra stop for the methane production which would bring cheers and respect from tough seventh graders every-where. But I am twenty years old now, nearly two and half years into my colitis experience, and feeling grim about the whole thing. That Bugs Bunny telephone booth plunges off the cliff and I cannot open the door to step out onto safe ground.

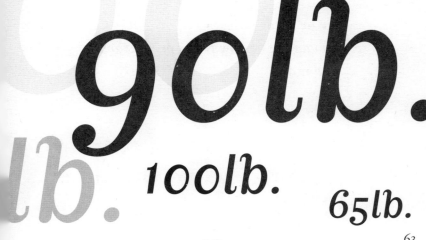

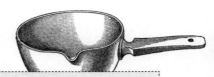

date:
5/17/1992

days since diagnosed:
900

age:
20

weight:
162

location:
ithaca, ny

medication:
occasional advil for back,
unused sulfasalazine

general symptoms:
frequent b.m.'s (unformed or running);
bloated stomach after eating; occasional
blood in stool; "brain fog", back/hip
pain

diet restrictions:
no dairy, no raw fruits or vegetables,
no nuts

attitude:
mixed

stuc

GOOD GRADES

In the beginning of junior year Dylan and I continue to go to the gym. With my strength returned and believing I am doing everything I can regarding my diet, I continue to search for answers to my bad digestion. The gut's still no good, more gas than anything. I feel I need to do something else to reduce stress: I became convinced that if some Freudian linchpin can be pulled, everything will drop away, and I will become whole again. I tick through the list of what contributes to health or the way I "used to be": the strength is there, my diet, according to a nutritional analysis paper, is dead on perfect: the right mix of complex carbohydrates, protein, and almost no fat. But I used to do better in school, maybe not that much better, but until this year, my third year of college, I did not care. I "suddenly" notice that college is half over and that I better pay more attention to class. My apartment-mates study diligently each day; so does Dylan, approaching his course work with the same intensity as lifting. I need to do the same. I decide it's time to earn A's; then my gut will work properly again. I buy index cards, do my homework on time, and stop skipping so many classes, regardless of how useless they seem when living with a bad gut.

Halfway through the semester I blow my straight A's. It's one question on one labor economics test. I realize it with only a minute left. I want to kick myself. Back at the apartment no one is there. I crank up the music and do a set of 75 push-ups.

I end the semester with the gut not doing any better. In the middle of finals, with little sleep and daunting tasks ahead, it gives out. With study time at a premium, I eat more often in the apartment. Meals consist of rice and soy sauce as I try to remain with basic, supposedly stomach-friendly foods. But I see mucous and blood.

For a statistics final, I sit exhausted in the front row of an auditorium waiting for the papers to be passed out. People are arranged every other seat. As the woman to my right begins to sit, she lets out an "Ohh!" and passes out, right there on the floor. A couple of us go to her side including an experienced student EMT. Soon public safety arrives. But now the tests are out, the exam has started, and this woman is still lying there. Complaints come from the second

homework

exams

and third rows to get that body out of here – it's too distracting. At semester's end, I earn four A's and a B, but still no solid BM's.

In the winter I work a three-week internship at an insurance company in Hartford, Connecticut. At the warehouse it didn't matter if you passed wind, you could be outside, walking around or driving the forklift. But in a hermetically-sealed office building things aren't so free. In the morning I jog on my father's treadmill for half an hour in order to get the gas out – nearly poisoning myself in the closed room. This is enough to survive the post breakfast gas and cramping, but after lunch the whole thing starts again. I make a habit of taking afternoon walks in the chilled downtown air.

At the end of the internship in January, I drive up to a friend's winter semester which translates to an excuse to drink. After spending vacation in a tan colored cubicle, I happily trudge through snow from one party to another, not wanting to think. The drinking leaves me sick. I return back to school a few days later than everyone else – letting my body recover, letting the Rowasa do its work to hold back the blood stripes.

+   +   +   +

For the spring semester I do even better in my classes and continue going to the gym. Habits remain steady but there is no gut improvement. However, I experience my first exposure to "alternative" treatment when I injure my back while running. A friend applying to chiropractic college recommends that I try a chiropractor instead of going to a regular doctor who would simply prescribe pain killers. I read a book on the subject, how the practice of chiropractic started and what ailments it can treat. In the first visit the chiropractor adjusts my lower back, immediately relieving all pain. He shows me an x-ray of my spine and says how its curvature due to bad posture can be improved with several more treatments. Although I don't mention it to the chiropractor, I hold out hope that the adjustments may help with the gut. In the end my back pain goes away, but that's all.

RUNNING AWAY

It's built into the culture. You keep on trying, you cannot give up.
You may be desperate, on the edge, falling into despair, on the verge
of throwing yourself in front of a train but then, then you have to
kick yourself, pick up your head, shake it off, and make a plan to
escape, to move on, to give yourself a new beginning.

+   +   +   +

I'm in Ithaca, NY, over-looking Eddy Street from a half-empty
apartment with moving boxes strewn across the floor. Three roommates have left for the semester, another's out drinking with his girlfriend. As the printer churns out my last paper, I consume my staple
foods for final's week: rice and soy sauce. My gut already feels bloated but I am on my way to a good life. I came back at 4 a.m the
night before and I think I'm in love with a woman across the street.
But before I start a serious relationship, I have to heal my body. I
have great hope. I have tried medicine, exercise, following my high
complex carb diet, and studying hard in school. The only place to
heal has to be buried in my mind, some kind of psychological
screw-up I can't detect, some fear I have to face. After my paper
prints, I will be done with my semester and on my way to Alaska.
The plan calls for driving there with Frank's college roommates,
working ridiculous hours on a fishing boat, and returning with
money in my pocket, a fresh view on life, and no more sickness.

Over the past weeks I've lifted weights, run, and read up on the
fishing industry – including using accident statistics from the
Alaskan Department of Labor for a class project. Frank's roommates,
Ed and Mike, complete their own training. We read that 48-hour
work stints are not uncommon for some types of fish openings.
Ed and Mike attempt 48 hours of non-stop activity. Following a
Friday of classes, some drinking, and going out to parties, they
drive from Rhode Island to Vermont to go snowboarding. They
make it down the mountain but somewhere in their 37th hour,
while driving back to school, they collapse, pulling the car over to
the side of the road and falling asleep. In high school, Mike lived
in Vermont and one year won every event in the state swimming
championships. Ed's a college sprinter and plays soccer. He weighs

210, is built more like a football player, and keeps a maim list on his wall – names of people whose bones he's accidentally broken during soccer games. I don't meet either of them until the day of the journey.

Ed drives up to North Haven, Connecticut, from his parents' New Jersey farm in a gold spray-painted VW Beetle. My parents don't understand my need to go to Alaska and watch in confusion as I throw my Army surplus duffel bag in the backseat, get into the car, and... go nowhere. The car will not start. Ed, myself, and my family push the vehicle up a slight incline and down the driveway before the engine catches. We don't shut the engine off until we turn into Mike's driveway in Maine.

There we meet and transfer everything to Mike's Jeep Cherokee. The plan was to go to Costco to buy food for camping. Food is my main concern for the trip and key to my gut making it so far. I still avoid vegetables, fruit, and milk products including whey. Both Ed and I want plenty of pasta. But Ed looks in the back of the Jeep and shakes his head.

"Mike, what's all this food?"

"I went shopping before you guys got here so that we could get an early start."

Ed picks up a can of asparagus spears and slowly turns it – studying the unappetizing picture. He examines the other cans.

"What's this?! Asparagus Spears and Beenie Weenie! That's what we're going to live on this summer!"

"It's only for the drive over there."

I spot a couple of packages of small cereal boxes – those single serving sizes they have in diners. I can survive on those.

+   +   +   +

In one week we have a ferry reservation to travel to Juneau from Haines, Alaska. We decide to drive to Haines in eight hour shifts.

Two people sit up front and a third sleeps on an air mattress in the back. We make it to Minnesota in the first twenty-four hours without incident except for the collapse of the air mattress.

By the time we reach Juneau my back pain returns. I think it's somehow connected to my gut. I eat twice as much as Ed and Mike – both of whom weigh at least forty pounds more – and I still feel hungry. At one stop I try slow jogging to loosen up my back but it doesn't work.

+   +   +   +

In Juneau we set up camp in view of a glacier and a mountain. Picturesque but similar to living by a giant ice cube – I wear a wool hat all the time. In an attempt to get fishing jobs, we walk the docks. Ed wears dark green rain gear, well worn from use by his father – a rugged, 300 pound wildlife enforcement officer. Mike has twenty year old gear from his parents' many sailing expeditions. I'm stuck with my cheap sky blue rain gear – the only stuff left at Sports Authority before we began the trip. I ditch the gear, throwing on extra flannels and sweaters instead. There's not much work until the next month.

Ed gets a Halibut job which means he'll be gone for four days. Mike and I spend a day baiting long lines in exchange for beer. We decline an offer to work on a rickety fishing boat with no safety gear. Instead Mike wants to hike the mountain close to our campsite. My back pain, exacerbated while standing and baiting has increased, making it difficult to walk on flat terrain. However, I haven't mentioned any health concerns – neither the gut nor the back. Mike and I don't have much to do, so I grit my teeth and make my way to the mountain with him. At the base, search parties fan out to look for a hiker lost several days before. After the first two hours of the ascent, I find my back doesn't hurt each time I put my foot down. The action of lifting my knees high and pushing myself upwards may be done without pain. As we continue I feel myself getting tired but I pretend I'm some kind of superhero, a blob: I picture myself rolling up the hill and keep up a strong lead pace – not really there, just rolling up the mountain.

We reach the top several hours later and create a new path down.

alaska

By the end of the day my spinal column is back in line and my body partially restored – but digestion remains the usual bloated gas affair.

For his several days of work, Ed makes a quick $1,000 and keeps muttering, "I could have died. I could have been seriously hurt." Mike has some savings, but I'm fast running out of money. The salmon fishing season won't open for another month so I take a ferry to Ketchikan where employment opportunities seem better – a cannery is hiring the following week.

+   +   +   +

I'm wrapped in a mummy bag, cocooned in a lounge chair on the back of an overnight ferry to Ketchikan. Passengers gather along the railing by the edge of the boat. They point at the sea and talk as the captain announces "3'o clock!" "6'o clock!" "4'o clock!" People shuffle as he calls out the positions of whales which move all around the boat. But I'm interested only in food. I have a small stove in my bag, and a box of rice. I have no place to legally light the stove and no cash. The owner of the chair to my right, a backpacker, stands at the railing. I'm eyeing the bag of granola beneath his seat. If I could reach a bit farther... But I don't move, instead I turn my head back and close my eyes. When I wake up the people to my left start chatting, and offer me food. At the next stop I make a trip to the bank.

+   +   +   +

Tongass Highway. Only minutes off the ferry. A stream of cars and trucks makes its way off the boat, friends and relatives pick up walk-on passengers. A flurry of late night activity and then everyone is gone. With a map and vague directions to a youth hostel several miles away, I begin the trudge with a big army bag strapped to my back and a smaller duffel bag in right hand.

On the drive up through the Yukon, Mike, Ed, and I stopped at a lake which stretches to the horizon. No sign of human activity. After fifteen minutes of staring silently at the lake, Ed spoke.

"Too bad we don't have a boat."

Mike surveyed the thick tree branches on the ground and small trees by the shore.

"I have rope. We can build a raft."

Armed with a small hatchet, we spent the next six hours cutting, bundling, blistering, and willing a small craft into existence. We each sang to ourselves to keep going – something from the CDs on the drive up. For me, "Sixteen Tons" had stuck in my head. I kept on singing and kept on going.

Now, making my way on the road to the youth hostel, slightly off balance due to the duffel bag in my hand, I begin singing the song again:

> Some people say a man is made outta mud
> A poor man's made outta muscles and blood
> Muscles and blood and skin and bones
> A mind that's weak and a back that's strong.
> (Tennessee Ernie Ford)

As I start the second verse, I turn to see a woman driving next to me in a van, watching and shaking her head. I stop. So does she.

"Do you even know what you're doing?"

I say nothing, embarrassed by my singing.

"Well?! Do you?" She laughs.

She gives me a ride to the youth hostel. I thank her and walk up the steps to read a sign informing me that the facility's closed for the night. I sit on the top step, lean against the wall, and fall asleep.

+   +   +   +

In the morning, waiting in a job applicant line for cannery work I meet Aladdin, Joe, and Zeke. Aladdin's half-Egyptian, same complexion as myself. Zeke and Joe are from Zimbabwe but have been living in D.C. for the past few years. Aladdin drove up from Illinois in a battered Datsun, and after we hand in our applications and complete interviews, he offers me a ride to another cannery which is signing up workers. However, similar to the first place, no one's starting operations for another four weeks.

With the youth hostel beyond everyone's budget and campgrounds miles out of town, we follow a tip and make camp in the woods at the base of a mountain, directly behind the Bay View cemetery. The town lets people camp here for the summer but clears the place out at the end of salmon season.

+   +   +   +

Maps mark the woods here as rain forest. We spend the next day in the library as the camp gets drenched. There's not an empty chair around. The vagrants have landed. The librarians make their rounds, prodding people, telling them if they fall asleep they'll have to leave. Aladdin rummages in the Datsun, below the leopard skin seats and letters from his girlfriend and pulls out a chess set. I'm a decent player, I beat all but one person on my first-semester hallway. But Aladdin, his forearms oversized from boxing and covered with welts from mosquito bites, makes his pieces fly across the board, destroying me every game – playing at a different level.

+   +   +   +

Tatsuda's Market is a short walk down the road. If we don't cook, we buy meals there, going an hour before closing time when they mark down the lunch food before throwing it out.

+   +   +   +

Zeke, Joe, and I find jobs at Sea Mart Supermarket. I'm in the shipping department which means writing down phone orders, taking a cart to go through the store to shop the order, boxing the stuff up so it's fit enough to take a ride in a sea plane (which is how many orders are eventually delivered), and sending it off in the supermarket van. The job requires wearing a white button-down shirt and a Sea Mart tie. It means shaving and getting cleaned up each morning. Most of the laundromats have token-operated showers. The laundromat next to the cemetery costs too much but there's another laundromat, shortly after the supermarket, where the cold water works for free.

vagrant

```
date:
```
7/17/1993

```
days since diagnosed:
```
1,320

```
age:
```
21

```
weight:
```
152

```
location:
```
bay view cemetery, ketchikan, ak

```
medication:
```
occasional advil for back,
unused sulfasalazine

```
general symptoms:
```
frequent b.m.'s (unformed or running);
bloated stomach after eating; occasional
blood in stool; "brain fog"; back/hip
pain

```
diet restrictions:
```
no dairy, no raw fruits or vegetables,
no nuts

```
attitude:
```
ignore it and keep going

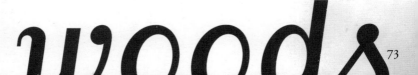

The mornings start off with a short walk to Tatsuda's for a box of Pop-Tarts which contains about 1,600 calories. I'm losing weight so I hope the extra calories help. I finish the Pop-Tarts halfway through my 45 minute walk to the cold shower. I turn on the water, run in, turn it off, soap up, turn it on again, and rinse. I put on my white shirt, jeans, belt, tie, and boots, then head to work. Excess methane production works itself out on the walk. I focus on the sound of my footfalls, ignoring gut pains. If you keep moving, it can't catch you.

For lunch I buy something in the supermarket and eat it out back, sitting on the rocks by the sea. Afterwards I take a quick trip to the near-abandoned loo in the mall attached to the store.

In practice, the walk home lasts longer than 45 minutes. I travel with Zeke, Joe, and Aladdin. Stop at bars. We meet up with people in town, people from the woods, from the hostel, from the library. Co-workers at the market sometimes stop to give us rides.

+   +   +   +

I've moved from Mike's five-man tent in Juneau which had standing room for ten to a two-man tent consisting of a dome to cover my upper body and a sleeve to slide my legs into. My bed consists of plywood, an air mattress, and a thin but super-warm synthetic sleeping bag. The air mattress pops after a week and each morning I wake up with knots in my back. It begins to iron out by the time I get to work. The walk helps the back, but not the gut. Early morning trips to the laundromat rest room become the norm. In emergency situations there's always the woods.

+   +   +   +

I'm walking back from work. Three women driving a pick-up truck stop and invite me to a party. I hop into the back. They're of mixed Native American and white blood. We drive a few miles out of town, turn off on a dirt road, go past a big totem pole, and stop at an area with mostly trailer sized homes plunked down in the middle of scenic Alaska.

We go into a bigger, one story house. The room's filled with smoke and there's an older guy, perhaps 50, drunk, short hair, wearing inexpensive sturdy glasses. I see a picture on the wall with him in a Navy uniform. The women who picked me up have abandoned me. The guy in the chair sees me, the newcomer, and sits up scowling.

"Who are you? What are you?"

I tell him I'm Indian – from India. He relaxes and shakes my hand, "You Indians are OK."

He offers me a beer which I take.

I see a couple of babies, one strapped into a car seat and positioned on the edge of a coffee table. No one seems to notice it. Everyone's drinking, talking. I find myself listening to a guy going on about the importance of tattoos. He's been getting them every couple of weeks.

"Ever since my wife died in the house fire last year..."

There's shouting in the next room. Someone lets out a roar. I turn in time to see an Indian, who's sitting down, clench his hands together, raise them like a wrecking ball, and bring them crashing down on the kitchen table, breaking it in half.

People are yelling at him about their spilled drinks, now telling him to calm down, now laughing.

The three women who gave me a ride are bored. They're going back into town. We're in a car now, three of them in the front and me in the backseat. I know their names: Darlene is the pregnant one, the one who first asked me if I wanted to go to the party. Sheila, who's driving now, is about 22 with two kids at home. The third woman, Kim, is 16 and curses nonstop.

They pick up a guy on the sidewalk, a friend walking down the street. Ignoring the gut, I take a long gulp out of the Mason jar they're passing around and sit back. The new guy shows me a set of nunchucks he has tucked into his jacket. I'm nodding, telling him "pretty cool."

"Yeah, I got a good deal on 'em."

He's sticking his head out the window and yelling to cars. Now he's sitting on the window ledge. We're going about 40 mph. Now he's gone.

"What the fuck?" Sheila's pissed. "Where the fuck did he go?"

I gesture toward the window and shrug. "Out."

She pulls the car over. When it stops he re-appears, slipping back in through the window.

"What are you doing? Where were you?"

He smiles. "I was surfing."

"Get out of the car!"

"But–"

"Get out now! Now!"

We continue. I'm the only one in the backseat now. We pull up to a guy on the street with waist-length hair. He's wearing black jeans and a black mesh shirt. He looks pissed. I recognize him from another night at a bar. Clint. He's a local drug dealer. Bad news.

He and Darlene, the pregnant woman in the passenger seat, continue an argument from earlier in the day. I realize it's Clint they've been looking for. It's his baby.

Clint walks within arm's reach of the car. Sheila pulls up a few feet.

"Bitch!"

We're starting to pull away. Darlene's yelling now, getting the last word in.

"Well, fuck you! I've got a new old man now!"

She turns her head to indicate me. I'm startled out of my Mason jar state.

"What?!"

Clint looks at me and then Darlene. He lunges toward the car but we take off, back to the trailers.

I'm standing in a small trailer with four other guys, including the one who broke the table. Aside from a few clothes, a small TV, and boxing gloves, the room looks bare. I'm telling them where I'm from, telling them I have nothing to do with Darlene and Clint. They know it, they're depressed about the argument and warn me to stay away from the whole thing.

I'm not sure if Sheila's coming back to give me a ride. There's a police car circling around trying to find a lost 15 year old who broke up with her boyfriend a few hours earlier. I'm ready to get out. I'm getting ready to start the long walk back to the graveyard.

I hear Sheila yelling outside. Screaming. Everyone piles out of the house. Sheila and the Kim are helping Darlene who's half crumpled over. She found Clint and he has punched her in the stomach.

We get into the car again. This time with Darlene and Sheila in the front, me in the back with the mouth. We speed to the hospital.

I stay with them at the hospital until morning. The baby checks out OK and I fit in a trip to a clean loo. Darlene asks for the police but when an officer arrives she refuses to file a report. The nurse looks frustrated but shrugs it off:

"It happens all the time."

No matter what time these trips back from the supermarket end, Zeke and I always get to work the next morning. We may feel tired, burnt out, but while everyone sleeps, Zeke starts us off on our proud march. "This'll make us stronger. Look at them all. Lazy!" We laugh. Stepping out of the world of academics and cubicles for a while makes my gut problems seem not so bad.

For the second half of my time in Ketchikan, I work in a cannery. I keep my "summer" residence in the woods and move into the cannery-owned floating bunk house barge where we sleep four to a room.

The job isn't bad, just repetitive. They supply good food, medicine, housing, even do our laundry. We work from 8 a.m. to midnight with one hour breaks for lunch and dinner. There are also three fifteen-minute breaks during the work day, the last at 9 p.m. They close the line down at 11:55 p.m. sharp, that way they don't have to pay for a midnight dinner except for the workers selected for clean up duty – and extra overtime pay. I make the cut for the last week, happy to eat the midnight meal.

My job on the line is easy. At the beginning of the line, the fish come off the boat and at the end they leave in cans. I stand by the conveyor belts before the lid machine. Four of us line up side-by-side as 250 cans go by each minute. We rotate tasks between being a "picker" or a "fixer." The cans stream in from the left. If bones protrude from a can or too much skin shows on top, the second person, a picker, pulls the can off. If you're standing in the first or third position as a fixer, you wield scissors which are used to tidy up the can. This means snipping the bones so they don't foul up the lid machine or flipping over the flap of skin, to hide the scales and show the pink flesh beneath. After the scissor work, fixers return the cans to the line. The fourth person acts as a back-up to the second person, picking any cans that are missed. Two additional people stand across from us in front of a parallel conveyor belt. If any cans are underweight or overweight, a pneumatic puff of air blows them onto the parallel conveyor before they reach us. The people across fix the underweight or overweight cans by adding or removing fish meat as appropriate. There are four can lines running, each one with the same scissor wielders and weight fixers on the end.

Things run smoothly until after dinner. Then people working the machine which puts the fish into cans get tired. If they don't position the fish correctly, more bones and skin appear on the top of the cans, forcing us to pull more cans off the line. At 8 a.m., the cans come by at 250 a minute. Twelve hours later the speed remains the same. By the time 9:30 p.m. comes, we pull so many cans off that we have to start stacking them. Some cans fall on the floor, and even the hulking "quality control" people who spend the day simply staring at us pitch in to help. By the close of the day I blink

and see cans, people next to me begin looking like cans, and I dream of cans.

The cannery work is bad on the gut. I start to see blood again and the back pain intensifies. I no longer have the long walks to the supermarket to stretch my muscles.

As the last week of August approaches, only days remain before the semester starts so I spend my earnings on a plane ticket home.

Alaska was supposed to strengthen the gut, clear the mind, be the final cure for ulcerative colitis. I arrive for the next semester before classes but days later than everyone else. I delay in order to let the gut rest up, let the pain in my back subside.

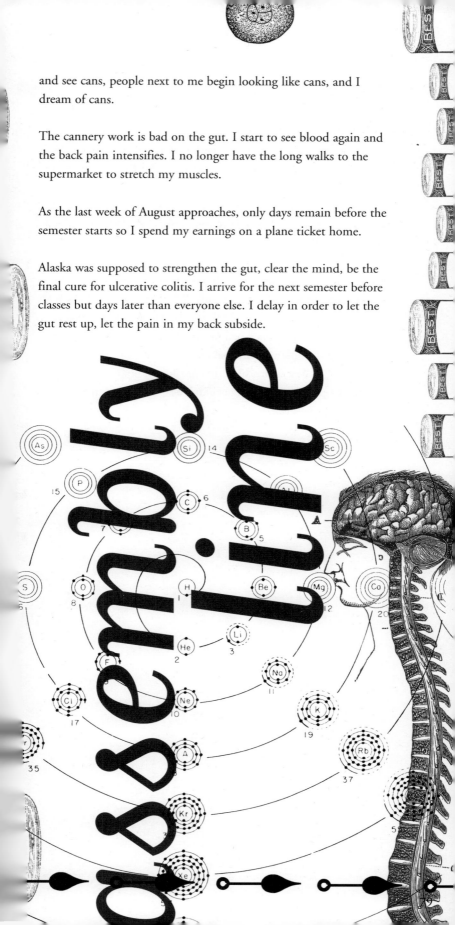

PRINCIPAL

My high school principal towered over the students. A Vietnam vet with a brief stint in the NFL and sterling academic credentials, he had decided to dedicate his life to education. When he came to our school he earned the respect of administrators and students alike. Years after my graduation, I heard that he had severe diverticulitis. After that I caught sight of him once in public. He looked haunted, ghostly, deathlike.

Months later he had a major operation. In the following weeks he began jogging to get his strength back. While he was on a back road near his home, a car struck and killed him. There was an article in the paper and things looked bad for the driver but then the story was dropped. I think my principal may have ended it. Right there. Not wanting to deal with a bleak life of surgery, pouches, and steroids. If a person that strong couldn't deal with bad intestines, I don't know how I can.

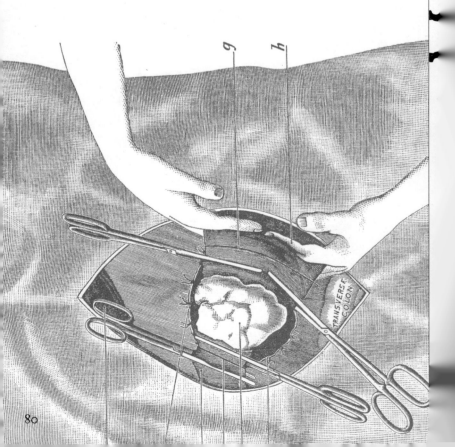

FRUSTRATION

I spend the next semester in Washington, D.C., working at a four-day-a-week internship at a Superior Court Building and taking a class. The University owns a building in D.C. with classrooms on the first floor and apartments on the floors above. We are 70 college junior and seniors living in doubles and triples. Freed from the cold and isolation of upstate New York, we have the energy and excitement of first-semester college students.

Workdays start with push-ups and sit-ups. Afterward I consume a packet of microwaved oatmeal, straighten out my shirt collar and tie, and head for the metro. By the end of the four-block walk my stomach starts bloating. I can't figure out why. Am I afraid of work? Am I going crazy?

By the time I get to work it isn't so bad. Officially I intern for the D.C. Mediation Service located inside the Citizens' Complaint Center. The D.C. police receive a million calls a year. The crack epidemic remains in full swing and the city's still thought of as the Murder Capital of the Country. With so much serious, violent crime, the police refer many "lesser" calls to the complaint center.

Depending on the nature of the complaint, the center issues restraining orders, schedules sessions with a social worker, or sets up cases for mediation. As an intern, I conduct intake interviews, determine where cases should go, and write up reports. The cases differ day to day, week to week. A vendor with a damaged cart: "I pay him to tow the cart back to the garage each day, he crashed it into the curb, breaking the axle, and refuses to pay for repairs." A 70-year old grandmother: "I'm older now. He breaks into the house, breaks windows, breaks locks. He's taken my TV, my money. But because he's my grandson, the police won't do anything about it." Neighbors fighting: "She's up all night banging around up there, banging on my head. I can't sleep. I don't know what she does up there but I need to sleep. I go to work early." The well-dressed, beautiful graduate student with a cast on her forearm: "He pushed me down the stairs. He says he won't do it again, he lost his temper. He's under a lot of stress. But he says he loves me." Visitation rights: "I don't want to sleep with my ex. I only want to see my

son."Occasional crazy people, including people my age: "They're
sending the subway to kill me. I have 26 children and 12 chickens..."

There are 2–3 love triangles a week of every type, of all ages and
sexual orientations. Many harassment cases come in, most of the
"I still love you and call you every night" type as opposed to the
"I stand outside your house every day and I want to kill you."
But those also exist. One woman is kidnapped by her husband in
the parking lot of her office. That afternoon he ties her up, beats
her, rapes her, and throws her back in the parking lot. During her
interview, he comes into the court building looking for her. He has
a shard of glass shaped like a knife hidden in a cigarette pack. The
guards find the glass-knife and arrest him.

Working there, we joke all the time. We have to. We're part of the
bureaucratic receiving end of misery. Some days it feels good to
work there, other days it makes me cynical. I walk around some
poorer neighborhoods, disillusioned, wondering why there aren't
protests or riots every day.

I sometimes jog in the morning in an attempt to relieve back
pain. Once I take a path in the woods bordering the sidewalk.
After a few steps in I suddenly jump, narrowly avoiding a sleeping
person. As my eyes adjust to the dawn, I see he isn't the only one.
Dozens of bodies lie sleeping, tossing with nowhere to go. The
city's a disgrace.

I work out, drink too much on the weekends, and live off the
energy of the "dorm" environment. I struggle with my gut and
soon establish my network of extra loos: loo on the first floor of
the college building, loo upstairs in the court building, loo at a
museum across the street from work.

Next to the court building, sitting in the fallen officers' memorial
by stone-carved lions on a sunny clear day, I eat from a styrofoam
carton of Thai food from down the street. It's better than the three
corn-dog special in Alaska, better than the cafeteria food in upstate
NY. I'm halfway through, just watching, appreciating the sky, the
people, my life. I'm four years away from my first bout of colitis,
from being on all the meds, spaced out, doubling over, that knife-
in-the-gut feeling. I finish up, toss the carton in the trash can,

knife-in-the

traight

and head back to work. The bloating starts now and the fuzzy-headed feeling – brain fog. There's some pain, but I stiffen my shoulders: Chest out. Gut in. Stand straight. Ignore it. March on. It'll make me stronger to endure. Eventually it will cease to bother me. It has to.

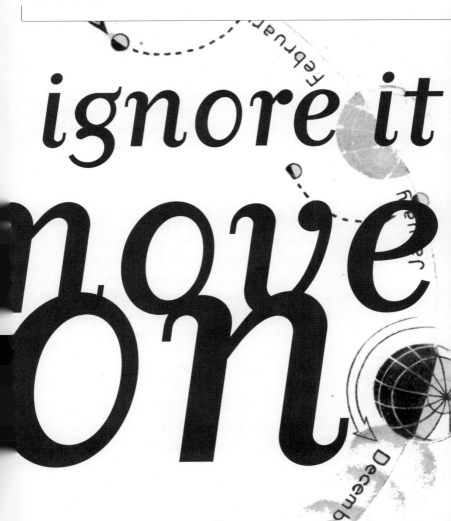

ignore it

move

on

endure it

feeling

FADING

The end of college passes in a fog. My health goes downhill.
The pain in my gut and hip persists, putting me in pure survival
mode. Despite lifting, stretching, and biking, I cannot get the
kinks out of my back. For the last semester I rent a single room
in a shabby house near the center of town. The floor tilts, buckles,
and curves. If I leave my chair anywhere in the room, it rolls toward
the center as if caught in a whirlpool. I share a bathroom down the
hall with two other people. No one spends more time than needed
in the house. My former roommates share a house with members
of the women's soccer and lacrosse teams. I originally had a room
there, but during my fall semester in D.C. I sublet to another
friend. He wanted to stay on in the spring and I consented. By then
I had no control over my gut.

I continue to eat in "athletic" proportions. Eighty percent of my
diet consists of complex carbohydrates; most of the rest is protein.
My gut produces enough gas to put me in competition with a cow.
I gave up a house which throws parties every week for a dilapidated
room in order to have bathroom privacy. But I have my ladder for
stretching and my Alaskan wool hat for when the heat fails.

+   +   +   +

I exist in a haze, continuously moving in order not to think or
take notice of what goes on in my gut. Walking from class to class,
I keep the Walkman on. Two nights a week I take a Wing Chun
martial arts class which doesn't involve high kicks or otherwise back
straining movements. The class never has more than 10 people and
leaves me relaxed. Afterwards I go to the cafeteria and get a late
night dinner consisting of two turkey sandwiches and potato chips.
I prefer being alone, traveling with my Walkman on and a book in
my bag to accompany dinner. The period after Wing Chun, ordering those sandwiches and chips, and sitting down to read provides
an oasis, a time to linger, a time to feel all right before the food hits,
the bloating begins, and the fog returns.

Relief from a gnawing gut comes after periods of exercise. Two to
three times a week Dylan comes in the morning to drive to Ithaca

Fitness Center. Throughout the semester the routine continues: the belt worn to protect the lower back, sweat pants, shorts underneath, a T-shirt. The day begins by shocking tired stiff muscles, stretching them, lifting, getting the body running again. For the next hour my head clears and I'm OK. Then I shower and go to class, picking up two cinnamon-raisin bagels with butter on the way. According to colitis guidelines given by the doctor, raisins aren't good for digestion. But plain bagels don't seem to be any better. I need the food but after eating, pain follows. By senior year I have my post-eating loos well marked out, stopovers for a lot of gas and some mucous.

I find it hard to concentrate while studying. The gut always made it tough but now I don't care. I don't see any long term benefits to the studying. There's no way to sustain living like this each day, trying to blast through the pain, hoping for it to just go away, for the gut to heal. The only thing that seemed to work was steroids and I've decided never to take them again.

I'm angry most of the time, wanting to put my hand over my gut in Napoleonic mode but instead clenching my teeth and walking on. I find solace in hanging out and drinking. The mornings bring intestinal disaster: seeing blood again, but the hours of relative happiness make it OK.

+   +   +   +

One weekend I visit my 1st semester college for a party. I convince three people to rent a car and pick up two others from Binghamton. I drive all the way down but when we arrive, the party's cancelled. I visit another friend at his frat party. Running and sliding across the floor, trying to do splits, trying to impress some girl and making a fool out of myself. Finding some basement loo, shitting all sorts of blood. Feeling a sense of panic and then saying fuck it!! My body's not any better off than it was four years ago. Go upstairs, grab another beer. Feeling loose and good, determined to overcome it all with pure enthusiasm. I keep drinking and dancing until the hundreds dwindle to a dozen.

At dawn, I find everyone and we decide to go back. There's still time to return the rental car within 24 hours and avoid being charged for another day. Two of us agree to stay awake for the first half of the trip and I take the wheel. My stomach's bloated, exploding. I unbutton the top of my pants. I focus on watching the road, sweating, trying to ignore the pain. Six hours later I arrive safely at my rooming house, at an almost private loo.

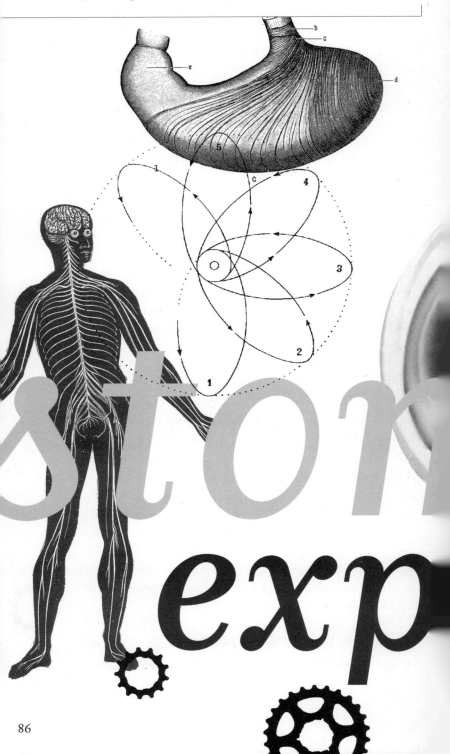

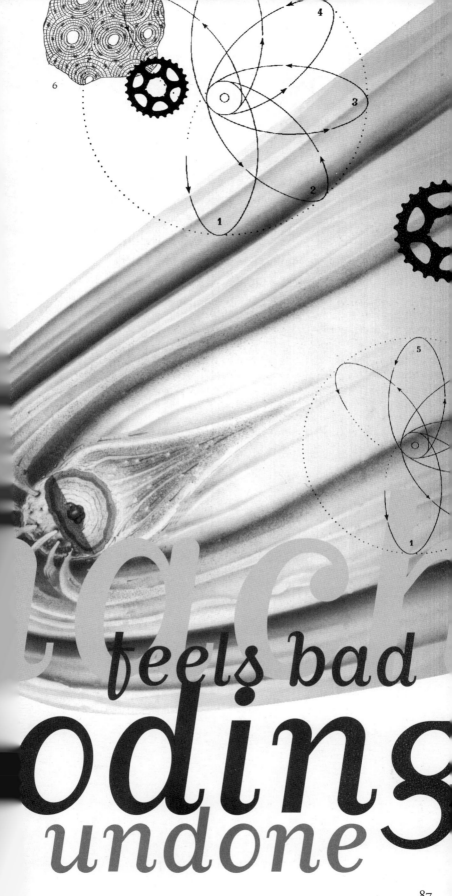

feels bad
oding
undone

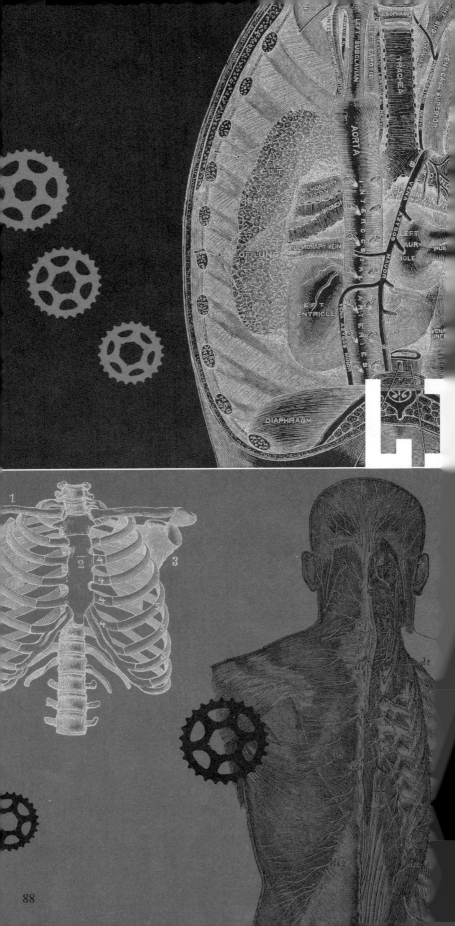

ESOPHAGUS
TRACHEA
LEFT SUBCLAVIAN
VENA CAVA SUPERIOR
INTERNAL
CAROTID
AORTA
INTERCOSTAL
VENA AZYGOS MAJOR
CUT
SURFACE
PULMONARY ARTERY
BRONCHI
LEFT
AURICLE
PUL
OF LUNG
PULMONARY VEIN
LEFT
VENTRICLE
VENA AZYGOS MINOR
INTERCOSTAL ARTERIES
VENA
INFE
DIAPHRAGM

1
2
4
4
4
4
3
5
5
5

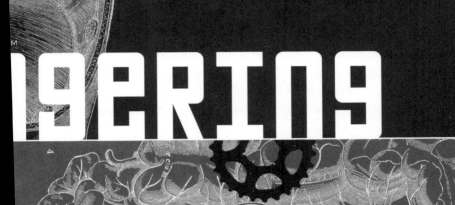

SURFACE
OF LUNG

SMALL   INTEST

ngering

MORE SCHOOL?

People are getting their post-college lives together: walking around in suits on their way to interviews, receiving the results of grad school applications, making plans for summer trips before jumping into the next phase of their lives. I watch it all with envy, realizing that I have spent my college years simply enduring. I can't imagine having to work in an office environment with my gut. I tell the doctor that the loo trips are three times a day but they are at least double or triple that number, not to mention my methane production. I have heard about some power plants running on methane – maybe I could get a job at one. I could go in head-to-head competition with burning cow patties.

I take an indirect way of getting better by applying to post-baccalaureate programs where students spend one to two years taking basic science classes in order to apply to medical school. I don't want to do it but I see no other choice. I hope that along the way I learn something about the digestive system which makes life normal again.

I apply to three programs. The most prestigious school requires only a name and address: they let you take the classes and charge a hefty fee. The other two programs are much more competitive and geared to assist students throughout the process including helping to matriculate into their affiliated medical schools. A recommendation from my supervisor at the D.C. Mediation Center helps me get into a program in the Boston area. Through a friend I meet a potential roommate, and a day spent with the program coordinator inspires hope. The school program will help arrange part-time jobs in the city. I look at some apartments but the whole bathroom situation again seems daunting.

Graduation comes with my family driving up for the day. I borrow a car and follow back a day or two later. I'm done.

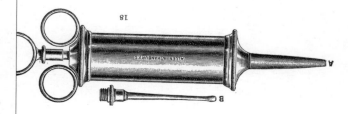

RAT LAB

One post-bac application, not due until after graduation, requires
research experience. A high school friend's father lets me assist in his
lab where they study the structures of the brain involved in post
traumatic stress disorder (PTSD). They are mapping out the brain
so the research may one day be used for treating people with PTSD,
such as war veterans. The lab uses buzzers and shocks to give rats
their own version of Vietnam. Once the rat receives "training," the
sound of a buzzer sends the animal into PTSD mode – pure panic.

For each batch of rats, they lesion (burn) away parts of the brain
in order to identify the structures involved in PTSD. If a batch
of rats with a specific part of the brain burned away goes through
training and does not show PTSD, then the researchers deduce
the burned away part of the brain may be part of the PTSD mechanism. It's a bit like the movies when cutting the right wire will stop
the ticking bomb but any other wire will blow everything up.
Except there are plenty of rats: if PTSD occurs (the rat "blows
up"), then they try another batch. By trial and error they map
out the neural pathways of the disorder.

A post-doc student patiently shows me the process of preparing
a rat: Grab it by the neck and swing it around a couple of times.
This temporarily stuns it, loosening up its muscles. Use a syringe
to administer anesthesia to the abdominal area. Place the rat into
a device which stabilizes its head: Hold the mouth in place by a
bar which clamps down on the overhanging front teeth. Insert rods
into the ears to complete immobilization.

Now the surgery begins. Cut the skin on the scalp and peel it back
to reveal the top of the skull. Wipe away excess blood. Use the ruler
on the stabilizer to find the center of the head and drill a hole to a
predetermined depth. Insert a thin straw into the hole. This straw
will be used to administer the chemical which lesions the brain.
Spread on dental cement to secure the straw to the skull. Staple the
scalp back together. Now the rat looks like it has a telephone pole
protruding from its head. Unclamp the sleeping rat, place it into
another cage. Go back to the other rats and pick another subject.
You have to be quick grabbing the second rat.

They see or sense the fate of the first and panic at the sight of your hand. After the rats have straws in their heads, they're allowed a day of rest before the shock sessions begin. Some of the rats receive chemicals which lesion the brain; some receive chemicals which have no effect.

I dislike the lab work. With the bad gut, I don't enjoy torturing the rats. In my first batch, one wakes up while still in the clamp with a hole in its head. Its body squirms while the head remains locked in place.

Once the experiment reaches completion, I kill the rats via lethal injection, putting them out of their misery. Next, I place them in the rat guillotine, dispose of the body, crack open the skull and make thin slices of the brain with what appears to be a mini deli slicer. I fix the slices of brain onto slides and examine them to verify that the correct places of the brain have been lesioned.

The lab is located near the Yale New Haven hospital and medical schools, plunked down in the middle of a run-down neighborhood reminiscent of D.C. In the morning I pull into an uneven gravel parking lot manned by a guard in a cheap polyester suit. The sound of the nearby highway grinds everything down. It's hard to separate my gut from my surroundings: the morning drive, the day of rat torture, and the walk back across the hot parking lot do nothing to boost my spirits. I feel all of it decaying.

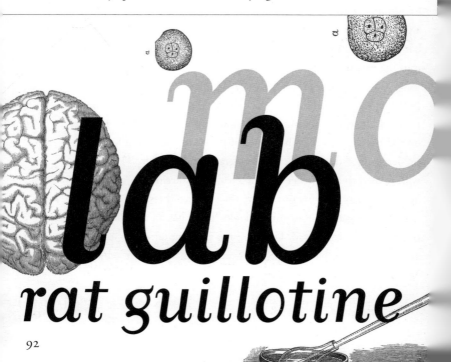

lab
rat guillotine

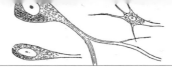

FAST FOOD

In ninth grade I ran the mile in track, four grueling laps. The races started fast around the first corner and never let up. By the third lap I didn't know how I was going to finish. But no matter how tired I felt, or how hard I was breathing, I could always kick and sprint for the last 100 to 150 meters. In soccer too, there was always some extra energy reserve that could be pulled out despite all exhaustion. Knowing it was there gave me a confident feeling. During college, I dug into this reserve almost every day, but at some point, it wasn't there. It disappeared.

I lose the angry momentum that kept me going through college. That anger fueled my vigorous exercise and strict diet. Working in the rat lab, burning the last of my savings (my paper route money earned between 5th and 8th grade), and living off my parents, I begin letting my diet slip. I still avoid milk products but I start eating fast food: the 99 cent Whopper signs prompt me to pull out two dollars every time. I splurge on Wendy's and occasionally I have the good fortune to pass by a Kentucky Fried Chicken restaurant. Flame broiled, "give me a double," extra crispy chicken and extra biscuits. As the days pass, the smell wafting from the fast food bags on the car seat next to me give genuine pleasure. I reason that since nothing seems to digest too well, why not enjoy the taste more. For 99 cents, who can go wrong?

+   +   +   +

You walk the balance beam with an ankle chain. A thick heavy chain with no way to remove it. You're walking in the dark. Moving slowly, trying not to rattle the chain, trying not to disturb the keeper, the monster at the other end – your bad gut materialized. If you slip, the keeper will awake and yank you back. Hand over hand, claw over claw, the monster will draw you down, beat you, bloody you.

You can't go fast: the chains will rattle. You can't slip: the chains will rattle. You will fall, tugging the chain, pissing off the keeper.

You think if you just eat "healthy," exercise, and do your work – live hard and clean – you will stay on the beam. But it's dark, you can

yank

keeper

see only a half-step ahead. The beam's not even straight. It dips, curves, and breaks. It narrows and widens. The beam has almost no thickness. It's flat. It twists and curves, ribboning out to nowhere.

Falling, stumbling, rattling, getting pulled back again and again. You attempt to go further each time, to learn the pattern of the beam. But it's not always the same: the beam changes, morphs. You fall, bang your chin. You begin to plummet but your chain snags. Dangling and dazed, you begin to climb back. A deep guttural sound comes from the other end of the chain. You're moving back quickly now, getting dragged.

But you try again and again to escape. Year after year, thinking you're getting a little further, thinking you're almost to the end. But no matter how far it seems, the beam doesn't end, the bloating is still there, the stripes of blood, the pain.

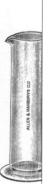

After high school, after college, you give up trying to walk the beam. You're bruised up from your attempts. It appears hopeless. You break this narrow thinking, this narrow diet, this exercise-no-matter-what mentality. You consume Burger King 99 cent Whoppers nearly every day. You tell yourself it's not so bad. You begin to settle in, sitting on that platform before the beam begins. You stop thinking about walking the beam. You stop thinking about getting out some day. You stop thinking about living. You hear that monster's throat rumble. You're being dragged in now! You'd better start fighting!

But you've been lazy, you haven't the strength...

+   +   +   +*gaun*

Between the stress, lack of exercise, and bad food, something in my body snaps. At the end of July, I indulge in a box of fast food chicken which ends in a bout of bloody diarrhea. The diarrhea clears and I return to the "normal," non-formed BMs, but I begin feeling feverish and spend a night puking. I eat lightly the next day, but I throw it up. A sharp pain in the upper abdominal area doubles me over. At first I think I've strained a stomach muscle, but I continue to vomit after eating or drinking.

emergency room

fading

HOSPITAL

It's 1 a.m. in the morning now. You sit at the kitchen table with the overhead light dimmed. Before you rests a glass filled with enough water for a mouthful. Elbows on table, head propped up by hands, eyes glassy, you look at the water, contemplate it. In the past hours you've tried a bit of ginger ale, a few sips of Gatorade, a half glass of water. Each time you end up kneeling over the toilet, yakking your guts out – the little bit of liquid and bile followed by dry heaves. You haven't kept anything down in over 36 hours. The mouthful of water represents your last hope. If you can't keep it down, you feel you'll just go to sleep and fade away. Pulling yourself up, you close your eyes, dreaming of water during half time at soccer games, of eating oranges slices, of standing under a waterfall. In your mind you're drinking it, dancing in it. It's reviving you, making you stronger.

You open your eyes, reach out and take the glass. You slowly pour the mouthful, letting it touch your dry lips. You put the glass down and wait. You will your body to relax. It's OK. You stand up and head toward the bedroom to collapse. But before you make it, nausea hits, and you end up back over the toilet bowl.

In the morning, you're forced to admit defeat. The doctor orders you to go to the hospital. The triage, the recitation of name, social security number, insurance number, address, and all information pertaining to your financial ability to complete this transaction. The waiting room, lolling. Entry to the emergency room. Stripping, putting your clothes, except for your boxers, into a bag. Slipping on the hospital gown, getting on the gurney, minimizing feet touching a cold tile floor. It's chilly, you don't weigh as much as you did a few days ago. The nurse brings over some extra blankets. You lie there, gaunt, half-listening, half-fading, trying to turn your mind off while you wait.

The nurse gives you an IV, they take blood samples, tell you they will be performing a stomach X-ray. Still you wait. Hours pass, you shift uncomfortably. You see a light-haired doctor in his mid-thirties looking at you. You note his European accent as he says something to a nurse. He turns to look at you. Eye-

dehydrated

to-eye. Mocking. He crinkles his eyes, perhaps mimicking yours. He gives you a street-acknowledging nod.

"Drugs?" he asks, smiling now.

You can barely speak. Something fires in your brain. Your unshaven face, brown skin: he thinks you're there for an overdose. What else can it be? You're too tired to be angry. Mustering your energy to speak your "best English," you tell him the exact problem, your doctor's name, why you're there.

He looks surprised but he reacts quickly, perhaps apologetically. Within ten minutes you're being wheeled up to a room, being checked in.

+   +   +   +

Dr. Brennan comes in to see how I'm doing. Not too well. I'm near tears when I see him. He takes a seat and explains the situation.

"Since it's Friday they won't be able to do much except take blood samples for more testing. I'm going to be on vacation but on Monday one of my partners, Dr. Sanderson, will look after you."

I'm on liquid drip so as not to get dehydrated. I share the room with a rotund elderly man who has a colostomy bag. He eats constantly, the hospital meals supplemented by his wife's home cooking. Every few hours the smell of the bag fills the room. An old man in the next room screams all night. He can be heard throughout the hall yelling: "NURSE, I CAN'T BREATHE!! I CANNOT BREATHE!" Every few hours the nurses come by to check my vital signs. Even without drinking anything, I end up dry-heaving during the night. This continues over the weekend.

+   +   _naus_

While Brennan appears neat, trim, and professional, Dr. Sanderson enters stomach first, a blaring red tie, an expensive shirt, the latest frames on his eyeglasses. He asks how I'm doing and schedules a panendoscopy where they snake a camera down your throat.

gaunt

On Tuesday my dad visits in the late afternoon, still dressed in his suit from the office. He asks me what Sanderson found with the scope. I tell him he hasn't come by. My dad asks the nurse to get him. Twenty minutes later Sanderson comes by. He says not all of the tests have come back so he didn't contact me, didn't bother to return several calls:

"I didn't see the point of calling if there's no news to report."

My dad starts speaking slowly, I can tell he's seething. He tells the guy that people should be told either way, not be left to wait for an entire day in the hospital.

My symptoms of nausea and vomiting continue. During the night, the nurse changes one of the IV bags while I sleep. Within 5 minutes, I wake puking my guts out again. She stops and looks at the bags. Twice a day they add a small bag of anti-nausea drug to my drip. She thinks it's causing me to vomit.

I've never been this weak. I can't read more than a sentence without losing concentration, fading. The bed becomes uncomfortable, my ribs jabbing into my skin.

I can get out if I can keep some food down, get re-hydrated. In the morning, a woman comes to draw my blood. I recognize her, Kari Cretella. Four years ago we shared the same high school cafeteria lunch table and we'd been in the same classes since elementary school. I'm thankful for a friendly face. She asks what's going on, what happened. I tell her about the nausea and inability to keep down water. She pauses, thinking.

"When I'm nauseous, I drink Sprite or 7-up and eat saltines. It seems to calm my system. I'll get you some during my break."

We talk more and I find out that she'll be starting classes to become a Physician's Assistant. When she leaves, I try to read, but my eyes begin blurring. I fail to finish a page.

weak

As promised, Kari comes back with soda and crackers. The saltines and stopping of anti-nausea medication seem to do the trick, or my

tears

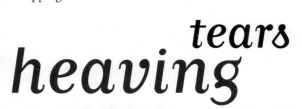

heaving

digestive system has received enough rest. After eating a hospital meal and not puking it out during the night, I am allowed to go home.

During my eight-day, seven-night visit to the hospital, not much is clear. They find a positive monospot. However, the main diagnosis is pancreatitis. In addition, the liver function tests return "mildly abnormal." A CAT scan of my gut as well as analyses of stool samples find nothing unusual.

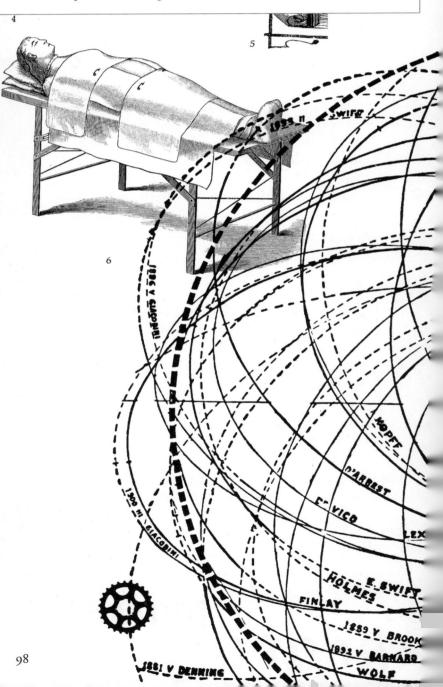

date:
7/30/1994

days since diagnosed:
1,693

age:
22

weight:
135

location:
hospital, new haven, ct

medication:
prednisone

general symptoms:
pancreatitis, upper abdominal pain,
frequent b.m.'s (unformed or running);
bloated stomach after eating;
occasional blood in stool; "brain fog";
back/hip pain

diet restrictions:
no dairy, no raw fruits or vegetables,
no nuts

attitude:
out of options, ignore it

LIGHTER

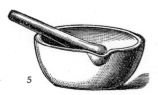

5

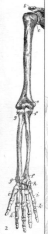

I arrive home weighing 135, a full 20 pounds less than before being admitted to the hospital. I feel chilled all the time and take to wearing a winter hat around the house in August. After I eat, the chills intensify and the fever returns. I feel as though I'll begin vomiting again. I find a solution, the barely used jacuzzi upstairs. It's a waste of water but getting in helps repel the chill, warms up my body, gets rid of the nausea, the shakes, the urge to wretch all over the place.

The reality of the weight loss hits hard. I stare dumb, disbelieving at the scale. The situation must be changed. Within two days, I force myself into the basement to re-tackle the weights. My arms struggle to curl and press. It takes more than the usual concentration. My legs and arms have atrophied from not eating and from lying in the hospital bed. I'm a skeleton working out.

I squeeze into the state university post-bac program. I'm hesitant about attending. I still have 10 pounds left to gain before my pants stay on again. I decide to start the program and rely on an uneven hole in my belt which I punched through with an awl.

The program begins hard. I approach it while ignoring my body, having the attitude of waking up after a late night in Alaska: "We will do these things because they'll make us stronger."

For the first six weeks of classes I commute 130 miles each day. I take chemistry, biology, calculus, and a writing class. My energy feels low but I make the drive, attend lectures and labs, and complete my homework. My body feels like shit. The gut aches, my back and hip hurt. In my classes people are starting fresh out of high school. I am in the advanced classes, similar to people I went to school with but I have few distractions, I only study and drive. Eating still bugs the hell out of me. I often eat lunch at a small Italian restaurant by campus. I order the spaghetti special which comes with a couple of decent meatballs and garlic bread. When I walk out I feel bloated, disgusting.

Because of the late acceptance, I send in all the loan applications for

atrophy

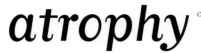

Central incisor
Late

weight loss

the following semester. After a month and a half, I borrow money from my parents to move into a small apartment for the rest of the year. My roommate is a physics Ph.D. student, a self-styled radical, peace movement guy. It's ok. In my room I sleep on a mattress on the floor. I set up my desk and note cards, and buy food I believe will get me through: oatmeal for the morning, sandwich supplies, and Rice-a-Roni for dinner. Not having to commute makes me happy, much more relaxed. I begin meeting people I knew from high school, now in their fifth years at the state university. I start a job watching over a small lab where I can sit and study. I go to the gym a few times and I do well on my tests.

For a while everything looks good: I make friends in my classes and have a small study group. But I am fooling myself, ignoring the pains coming from my gut, ignoring the times my stomach runs, ignoring any signs of blood, telling myself it's only tomato sauce from the night before.

In mid-November my roommate Steve comes down with the flu and I catch it. I spend a 24 hour period throwing up and having my stomach run. But I tell myself I am OK. The next day I have trouble keeping water down and my upper abdomen hurts. I fear the return of pancreatitis. No way. I am scheduled to oversee the lab that night and I go. Keeping my back straight, with Zeke, Joe, and Aladdin in my stride, I walk up the sidewalk snaking over the lawn to the lab building. Halfway there, nausea hits. I lean over and puke out the Gatorade I drank half an hour ago. My stomach heaves again. It is getting dark out, I straighten up, look around. No one sees me. I clean up a bit in the men's room, splash water on my face, rinse out my mouth. OK, no problem, carry on. I sit in the lab. With my science and math done, I work on a paper for my next writing assignment. A sole person uses the lab, an Indian-American woman carrying out an experiment. We talk and she lets it be known that she doesn't waste her time on things like reading or writing: they are stupid, not important. I shrug. Oh well.

The next day I am still not keeping anything down. I go to the school medical center. A no-nonsense older nurse sees me first. After I explain the situation she says, "You'd better find out what's causing this or you're in trouble."

remolar   1st molar   2nd molar   3rd molar

101

"But, how?"

Lips pursed, eyes hard, she speaks again: "You have to find out."

I'm pissed. I want to tell her off. How am I supposed to find out?! Didn't I already do everything I could think of? If it is not stress or diet, it's a goddamn mystery to me. If Brennan and Sacco and other great brains of science can't help, then how can I be expected to waltz out there to solve the problem! It's ulcerative colitis, lady! There is no cure! I say nothing. She pricks a nerve, she's right but I don't know where to look.

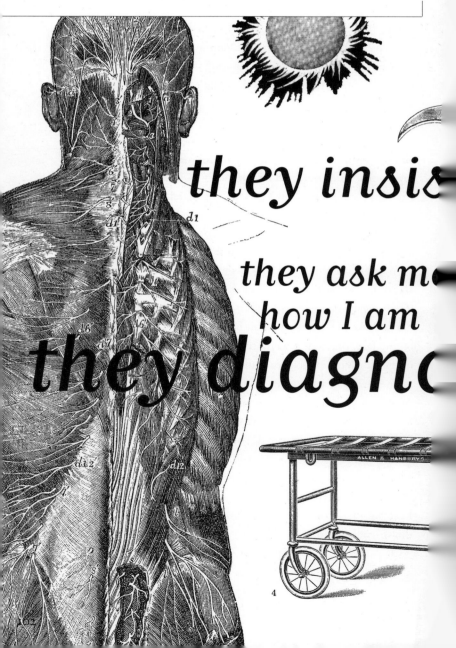

they insis

they ask m
how I am

they diagno

4

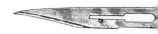

THANKSGIVING

With no liquid for nearly 48 hours, I try a few more times to keep water or ginger ale down, but fail. I use all my concentration to drive back to my parents' house. Right before Thanksgiving, I check in again at the hospital. The first night at the hospital I stand by a window, look several stories down, and decide to end it. One jump to stop my misery. Dropping out of the post-bac program, feeling like shit all the time. It's been going on for five years now. Five years! I can't get the window open – it's locked shut. I think of picking up a chair and trying to break through it. But there is a patio one story below – falling to the patio probably wouldn't do it. I go back to bed and fall asleep.

+   +   +   +

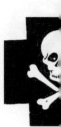

After that night, I receive a steady stream of visitors. My parents, my sister, my brother, my grandmother, aunts and uncles. Although I lose more weight this time, I retain enough energy to read. Between visitors and books, I try not to think. Instead I focus on my Tom Clancy novel. The book's main character leaves the hospital and gets his health back with a vengeance: running and lifting weights. Lying there with my rapidly disappearing body – legs tend to get thin quite fast in the hospital – I decide to do the same, and fall asleep.

They wheel me down for a barium test – where you swallow a glass of a thick chalky substance and they take X-rays as it passes through your digestive track. I tell them it's a bad idea. I'm in the hospital because I haven't been able to keep anything down. They insist. Halfway through the test, I ask for a tray to puke in.

They diagnose pancreatitis again and decide to send a scope down my throat to check for the cause of the vomiting. My gastroenterologist, Dr. Brennan, is on vacation so one of his associates carries out the procedure. Covered with three blankets I lie on the metal gurney in the center of the room. Medical instruments surround me. A nurse comes in and begins readying equipment, asking me how I am. I say fine, half mumbling, too weak to say much but

they wheel me down

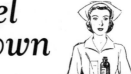

date:
11/28/1994

days since diagnosed:
1,811

age:
22

weight:
135

location:
hospital, new haven, ct

medication:
prednisone, azulfidine

general symptoms:
bloody diarrhea; vomiting, unable to
keep anything down; back/hip pain

diet restrictions:
no dairy, no raw fruits or vegetables,
no nuts

attitude:
negative

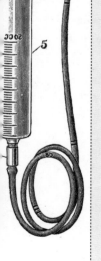

happy for her asking. A young doc comes in the room and begins talking to the nurse, reconstructing every delicious bite of his Thanksgiving meal on the previous day. I see the nurse shoot the doc a look telling him to shut up. He continues, "the gravy was made from—"

"Maybe we should talk about something else – he [the patient] spent Thanksgiving here."

The doc doesn't get the hint and continues onto the cranberry sauce. The nurse turns her back and does her best to ignore him: the man standing at the foot of my gurney, reciting food. As he starts on dessert, another nurse and the main doctor come in. The procedure consists of sticking a camera down my throat and stomach in order to look for any signs of disease. They'll watch a Sony Trinitron monitor while guiding the camera down. The nurse attaches anesthesia to my IV and uses a spray on my mouth in order to numb it. I begin to get sleepy as they place the camera down into my mouth. But I gag on it. I cannot breathe. I grab onto the tubing of the camera to pull it out. I see the eyes of the Thanksgiving day doc as he angrily grabs my wrist. At that moment I snap, deciding to get him. I move my hand in a small circle, breaking his grip and grabbing his wrist. The eyes widen on the faces above me. Three more pairs of hands descend, grabbing my arms as I black out. When I awake I am getting wheeled back to the room.

They don't find anything. But my voice has dropped to a whisper, the back of my throat bruised up from the scope. I imagine the Thanksgiving doc having a turn and banging the camera down my esophagus, making up for my grabbing his wrist.

They run a CAT scan and finally schedule an appointment with the dreaded steel stallion, the colonoscopy – during which they put you out the entire time. The scope shows severe intestinal inflammation and I return to the prednisone via IV. On my ninth day I keep down food and on the tenth day receive a discharge as well as prednisone and Azulfidine prescriptions.

I do not want to know where I am. I do not get along too well. I feel isolated, a bit ashamed. If I can ask for one thing, it would be to gain weight, simply put on weight. Leaving the hospital at 130 pounds, I feel my ribs when I lie down. In the car, I ask my mom to keep it slow: the bumps hurt, they jar my organs. There's no padding around them.

+   +   +   +

During December I do nothing but sleep, read, eat, and exercise, trying to gain all that weight back. I start with a small bowl of chicken and rice. Within minutes I feel chilled, my forehead begins sweating. I go upstairs to the jacuzzi, unused since my last hospital visit. I fill it up and sit until the fever begins fading.

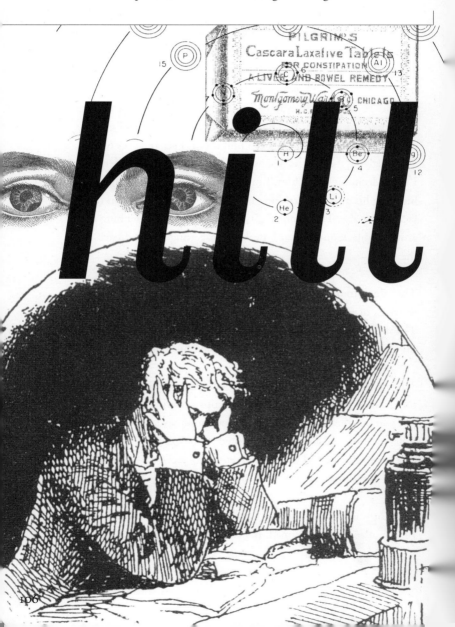

BASEMENT

The two places I spend the most time after the hospital are my parents' basement and the hill. Near the end of my senior year of high school my parents added an addition to the house which included an extension of the basement. The washer/dryer, furnaces, oil tank, hot water heaters, most of the house mechanics and extras were shifted to the new basement. It is windowless and reachable through another windowless room of the old basement. It's a dark room off a dark room – one of the few places offering privacy from the noise and clambering of other family members. Down there I set up a radio, desk, chair, and lamp. I shut the outer door by wedging the shoulder side of an old crutch under the knob. Sometimes I turn on the lamp light and read. Other times I crank up the stereo, Pantera or Guns 'n Roses, and write. Mostly madman stuff about race and hate, violent scattered thoughts on broken things including the state of my health. But most times in the basement I eventually head for the hill. I drown out any potential sounds with something quieter – a mixed tape or Seal or REM's *Automatic for the People* album.

I place my feet on the desk, lean back in the chair, close my eyes, and beam out of the basement, the house, the whole damn town. I drift to upstate New York in the summer to a place outside of the university where I used to bike. Off the main roads, on a hill, stands a tree. One of those out of a painting picturesque spots, a perfect shade-giving tree. I put my bike down on the grass, take off my shirt, and lie on it, face to the sky, eyes closed, feeling my muscles loosen and my body sink into the curve of the ground, the sun beginning to draw sweat from my skin. I lie there, sometimes thinking of a certain woman, but most of the time drifting. My body feels no pain after biking, adrenaline temporarily washing away all heath problems.

When the tape ends I abruptly return from the hill to the basement. I stumble to find the main lights, double back to click-off the stereo and weak desk lamp. Remove the crutch wedged under the outer door. Head out semi-peaceful. Another day gone. Hoping the next one will turn out somewhat better.

HOCKEY

As the year rolls around, the pond behind the house freezes. From the window I watch people play hockey. Winter used to be the best season. As soon as the thermometer dropped I'd run out before school to check the ice – run out with a ruler. Kick off a chunk of ice at the edge and measure it. Two inches was marginal – the ice may-or-may-not break, but four inches could support an elephant. Tige, my next door neighbor would also be out there. We didn't see each other much. We were in different grades, different classes. But each winter, as soon as the frost hit, we'd be by the pond, nodding to each other:

"How have you been?"

"All right."

"How's the ice?"

"Good."

We'd walk out on the frozen pond in our workboots. Stand in the middle, stomp on it a few times. We'd run back to our houses, returning outside in minutes. Sticks, skates, pucks. With an hour left before school started, we'd lace up as fast as we could and jump onto the pond, breaking in the new ice – black ice. The first ice of the season was clear. You could look down into the water. We'd go fast, gliding, floating across the pond, looking back at the white trails made by our blades. Passing the puck, huge shots, end-to-end slap shots.

When the pond froze, hockey came first. Homework never made it out of the backpack, after school activities ceased. Grades dropped. Hours of sleep decreased. By the second afternoon, word spread throughout the neighborhood. Joyce and Crouch. Robinson, Vercellone, Wolkovitz. The Villanos. Sometimes Arnold. A group of smaller kids with skates of varying quality and sticks taller than themselves. One big hockey game would begin and we would do our best to keep it going. If it snowed, an old piece of plywood, not seen in the warmer months, would magically re-appear. At least

rail thir

two people would push it, clearing out a rectangle. When we became older, in ninth grade, at least a few dads owned snow blowers. Family cars would continue to struggle through snow-covered driveways but the "rink" would be blown clear. Tige and I worked to keep it skatable as long as we could. A puck spray-painted orange, a step ladder, 100 feet of extension cord, and an ancient spotlight found in someone's garage kept us going in the dark. If too much "snow" built up on the rink from constant play-ing, we'd go out there with buckets of water and throw it on to try to clear off the ice – a slow Zamboni. One day, when the tempera-ture hit nearly 40, we all stayed off the ice – except for one pudgy kid who walked all over the "rink." Big, four inch deep footprints covered the area. We yelled at him, dragged out a garden hose, and spent the afternoon trying to repair the damage. The next day, when the temperature dropped, the rink was lumpy but skatable. We banned the kid from the pond for weeks. When the pond became solid, school and our parents faded away as we returned to the ice.

But that was years ago. I'm 22 now. Tige has moved. Even the small kids have grown up and left. I don't know anyone out there. My hip cracks. I'm rail-thin, sickly. I turn away from the skaters and head off to go read, in the dark basement room.

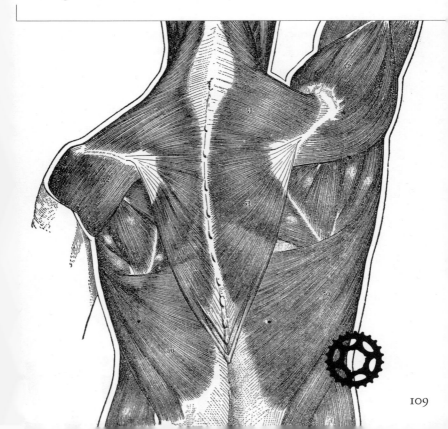

QUITTER [6]

I'm a quitter of vast proportions. I have quit soccer in high school as well as track and karate. I have lost the ability to run properly because of back pain. Quit the post-bac program, stopped communicating with most of my friends. I don't want to try anything.

I think about school, the hospital, doctors, living at home, my bad gut, and how to get out of it: take more prednisone (no way), kill myself (nope), just get away, walk away, maybe search out my dad's family in India and find some kind of cure – anything. But I am here, back where I started, trapped in the house, filled with late high school memories of being sick, going in circles. I've dented up my room good. Fists and elbows through sheetrock. I am getting down to a minimal level of prednisone and going nowhere.

I am looking for a purpose, something to keep me going, to fill up the days while waiting for my weight to return. The first glimpse of hope comes through the local public access TV station. Usually it features a computer generated, scrolling list of events. However, while flipping through the channels, I catch an interview with a local man who has recovered from a chronic pain condition. On TV the man speaks of a car accident where a drunk driver on the wrong side of the interstate hit him head on. The most serious injury was a break in the femur close to the knee. In addition, the tendon severed, flipping the kneecap. The leg failed to heal properly and generated pain 24 hours a day. The leg ballooned in size. The hair fell out. In the month before the car accident, the man qualified for a national bodybuilding contest and completed chiropractic college. The son of a truck driver, he had worked and struggled to finish school and save enough to start a practice. The car accident drained his savings and left him living in the cramped childhood bedroom of his youth using a surgically implanted morphine pump to get through each day. After two years and seemingly endless doctor's appointments, the man went to the Mayo clinic in Minnesota. There they weaned him off the morphine and helped him increase the range of motion in his leg even though, by that time, X-rays showed osteoporosis. After two months, they presented the option of amputation. At that point something snapped: he decided to get better on his own, no matter what. He spent nearly another two years rehabilitating his leg, brutally breaking through the pain barriers and eventually recovering enough to compete in bodybuilding again.

I meet the man in January. He graduated from Quinnipiac College, one town away. He is interested in writing a story of his struggle with the chronic pain condition Reflex Sympathetic Dystrophy. My mother teaches part time in the Quinnipiac English department and he has looked up her name in an attempt to find a ghost writer. My mother doesn't have any interest, but she suggests that I help.

He agrees and it gets me out of the house again with a purpose. Armed with a dictaphone and yellow legal pads left over from college, we meet regularly for interviews. He is in the process of starting his practice and moving out of his apartment. Every few days, we sit amid moving boxes for an hour or two. In addition to the interviews, I have his medical records and hundreds of pages of journals where he recorded his medications, weight, hours of sleep, and general mood every day during the course of his illness. The journals start sober and clinical, loaded with medical terminology from the fresh-out-of-school chiropractor. Later, they became crazy, filled with drawings, rantings, pictures of chains. During the years of his illness, he averaged only a couple of hours of sleep a night. For weeks he didn't sleep at all, passing days in a haze of pain and morphine. Compared to his experience, colitis seems like nothing. It has to be conquerable. quitter

Reading through and listening to the chronic pain story, I regain some of the spirit to get on and improve my health. I sign up at a gym and attempt to rebuild. I often find myself dizzy, on the bordering of blacking out. Exercise doesn't give the response it used to, the hours of comfort afterward, shocking the body into getting strong again. Instead, I become weaker and need longer rests.

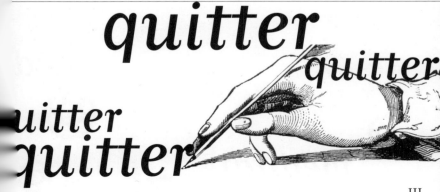

MEDITATION

For the chronic pain writing project I start frequenting the new Barnes and Noble, looking at similar stories of illness and recovery. I'm keeping an eye out for myself. Books on alternative medicine are beginning to hit the shelf and I'm ready to try anything. Nearly every book contains at least a paragraph on meditation. This prompts me to visit a Zen center in the next town.

The center is on the second floor of a well-kept house in a run-down neighborhood. Aside from the instructor, one other person attends the introductory session. The instructor, a lean, white-haired, middle-aged man explains it to me. He makes me suspicious, he looks too healthy, eyes too clear. He describes how the school and several others are based on the teachings of a Korean monk. The instructor, who has a full-time job with the state, says that the training doesn't involve martial arts. It also will not bring us enlightenment – he still hasn't had an "Ah-ha!" day where life suddenly becomes clear. Basically, each morning and night they practice an hour-long ritual. The first half consists of singing from a book of Zen-type chants. They are written in Korean so they make sense only if you look at the translations. The next half hour consists of meditation: Sit comfortably on a stool or pillow. Tilt your head forward. Fix your gaze on a spot on the floor. Let yourself breath from your belly – and allow your mind to clear.

The instructor describes the mind as a bucket of water with sand in it. Usually it is all stirred up, muddy. However, if allowed to remain still, the sand settles, things become clearer. But it's hard work.

"As you sit, you begin to think; one thought leads to another and soon you're off. The trick while sitting is that when a thought pops up, not to ignore it. Instead, acknowledge it. Let it drift away – a balloon with the string cut. Trying to force the thought away will only bring another."

"So you sit and cut balloon strings?"

"Something like that."

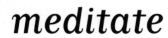

After an explanation, he asks if we'd like to try meditating for five minutes – just sit. We do it. Everything becomes quieter, a few car horns blare in the distance, someone shuffles in the adjacent room. But the space becomes new, peaceful.

I go back to a full session a week later where they sing and chant for the first half hour. Chanting in another language helps clear my head, breaks up my thoughts. The half hour of sitting is another matter. Halfway through, I become restless but stick with it. I leave clear-headed and feeling better—much better. I do more checking on the Zen center, it is Buddhist with no cults, monetary donations, or denunciations of the world required.

I go back a third time but at the end of the session I am angrier than I've ever felt. I don't know where the anger comes from but after that I don't go back: I become scared of going crazy.

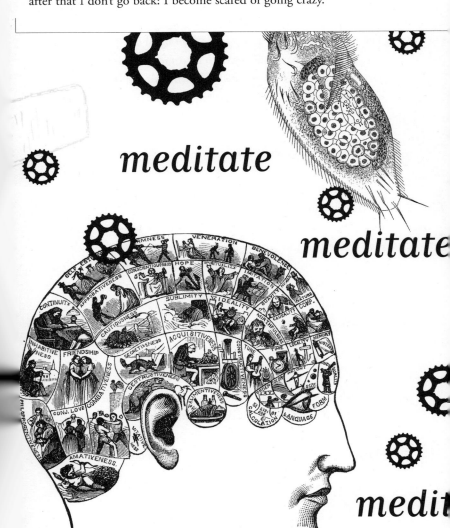

meditate

meditate

medit

MORE ALTERNATIVES

On another trip to Barnes and Noble, I buy a book which suggests eating bland foods for a week – only rice and chicken. After following this diet, the book describes how to add back one food at a time in order to test for allergies. In the end it doesn't help much. Even the rice and chicken diet doesn't settle my stomach enough. The dream of the solid BM remains elusive.

On another foray into the bookstore's alternative medicine section, I read an article on biofeedback – how patients may control "involuntary" functions. Perhaps by learning to control some aspects of my body, I will have a chance of better controlling the gut.

My last foray into this line of thinking came during sophomore year when I mail ordered a relaxation tape. Embarrassed that someone might find it, I copied the tape onto a blank and left it unlabeled. The tape made me fall asleep faster than usual but didn't yield much else. But biofeedback, there had to be something to it. If men could survive being buried alive, slowing down their respiration and bringing all processes to a near halt, surely I could have a proper bowel movement.

I decide to give it a shot. I see a small device in a magazine. For $50 I purchase a biofeedback unit that measures temperature. The instructions direct the user to tape the sensor to a finger and concentrate on making the temperature display increase. Back to the darkened basement, the lab. After a few sessions, I can raise the temperature in my hands but cannot detect any other changes. Within two weeks, the digital temperature display dies. The numbers cannot be read properly. Is it a 4, an 8, a 3? I can't tell. The biofeedback experiment stops and I toss the over-priced thermometer into a drawer.

+   +   +   +

While I was in the eighth grade, my father became wary of politics at work and the high cost of college education. As a backup plan, he convinced my mother to sink their meager but precious savings into buying and renovating a rundown mansion in New Haven.

My father made daily visits to inspect the contractor's work and help move it along. We spent every night cleaning up the work areas, hauling trash into a full size dumpster which was emptied each week. Old stoves, tiles, wood scraps. After a while of working in the dust, coming home at 11 p.m., and leaving clothes at the door, I began dozing off in math class. It was cool, fun, doing something "real" after school, real work. After the house was finished I helped maintain it for years: painting after tenants left, shoveling (and later snow-blowing in the winter), cutting the grass and trimming the hedges in the summer.

Now, with not much to do in the day, I take the pick-up truck and drive it to the house. There's always some lingering task to be done. It's strange now. I'm not so friendly, I'm not a school kid doing some odd work before going on with my life – this is it. Our family's never had a car as good as the tenants have. Most of them are near my age, bright graduate students. They always appear happy and healthy. I feel I've wasted my college time, but given another chance, I'm not sure if things would change. One thing I didn't do back in those junior high and high school days was use the basement loo, the secret loo which opens on the house's master key. I never needed to use it before, but now I have no choice.

+   +   +   +

The chronic pain writing project loses steam. The man's focus shifts to the myriad of details involved with opening his chiropractic practice while my head spins trying to figure out a way to get better. I want it all to work out like a movie. Neat and clean. You get sick, you suffer, you become healthy, you mature, and you go on again. After high school, I figured I would get better and walk out of it. Take the summer after high school to recover, start college new, fresh. End of story. The chapter would close, victory music would play, credits would roll...

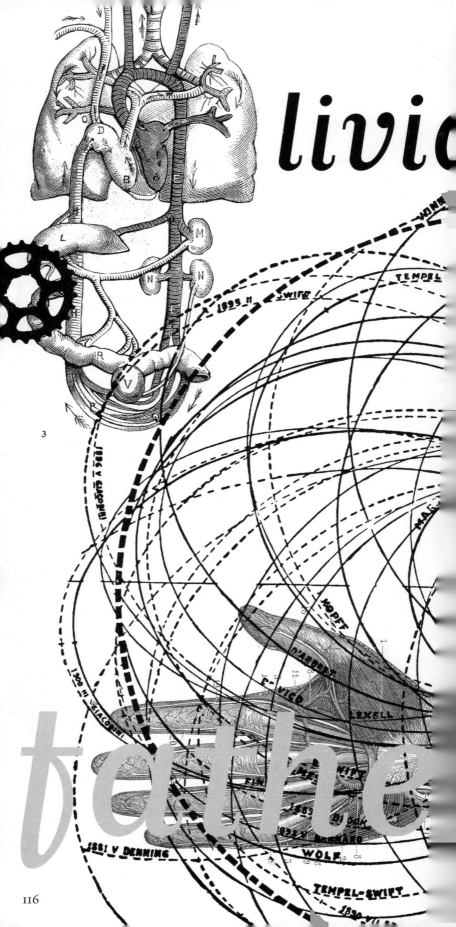

livic

fathe

PUNCHING WALLS

2,000 days with ulcerative colitis. When June and July come around, I remain so-so. Occasional blood, no meds, low energy. No plan. I busy myself back at the house. Make up things to do. Sweep this, paint that, straighten things out. I feel useless, a drain on my parents' finances but I'm not sure what else I can do. I have no skills and the gut remains in a perpetual state of misery.

My father is as frustrated with my being in the house as I am. He sets up a meeting with a friend of his from a consulting company. I wear a button-down white shirt and suit pants, and bring a resume. The friend gives me advice on a career and says his firm will contact me for an interview. I receive brochures describing the weeks of introductory training. Lying in bed, I look through the recruitment literature. Glossy pictures, the handsome, beautiful, and well-educated of every race having meetings, running on the beach, living in the best cities in the world. I mull it over. Eight life times have passed. I feel far from school or my D.C. internship, or walking down Tongass Highway in Alaska on the way to the supermarket. Consulting is serious work. With the gut still bad, not one good week, not one solid BM, I'm not sure how I can do it. There's no way I can do it. I already dropped out of a volunteer lab job and an academic program. Burning bridges, isolating myself. My body's in no condition for this Big Consulting Company.

My father gives me feedback on the Big Consulting guy's impression of me. GPA decent, good interpersonal skills. I tell him about the possibility of the interview. He looks pleased.

I write a thank you note to my dad's friend, but when a woman from the human resources department of the consulting company calls, I decline the interview. I don't want to fail again. I cannot predict how I will feel from day to day, so no way.

When I tell my dad I've declined the interview, he looks livid.

"You don't know what you're doing. Here's an opportunity to get a good job. And you blow it! You're wasting your life!"

wasting your life

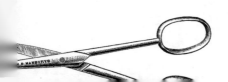

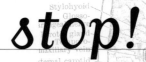

stop!

"My gut's still not good."

"I spend all this money on college. Wasted!"

His eyes become furious and he starts toward me, fists clench by his side. I back-peddle down the hallway, into my bedroom.

"He was doing this as a favor, just looking at your resume. I didn't expect him to set you up with an interview. It's not easy to get an interview at these places! And you just decline!"

"It doesn't matter because I–"

"What the hell are you going to do?"

"I–"

"What are you going to do?"

I haven't seen him like this since I was in junior high and swore in his presence. In that instance, he broke a three-foot wooden level over my backside. He takes another step into the room. I back up.

"What are you doing?! Don't take another step forward!"

He comes forward. I raise my hands up and put my right foot diagonally behind my left.

"Stop! Don't come any closer. I'm shitting blood all the time. Until that is resolved, there's no way..."

He isn't listening any more and when he moves toward me, I kick with my right. At waist level a large hole appears in the wall next to him – my foot smashed the sheet rock.

He looks at me, furious, confused.

He backs up. I kick the same spot a couple of more times. Crazy. I attack, opening up the wall with my foot and elbow.

He looks in disbelief and walks out of the room. I pause and follow.

wasted

I spent all

He is on the phone, dialing away.

"I'm calling the police."

As I walk by, he steps back. I go out the backdoor and into the garage. Taking out my bicycle, I head out onto the road.

With no plan, I end up less than a mile away at a high school friend's house. He is in the basement with two other guys, shooting pool and drinking beer. I hang out, tell them about the incident. They were good friends before college but I'm in-between lives, shaken, not trusting anyone. I stand watching the game, declining the chance to play, feeling too rattled to hold the cue. By midnight I hit the road again. With no place to go I find myself coasting under street lights. Miles of smooth pavement lined with sleeping houses. Quiet. I hear the sounds of the wheels on the pavement and the click-click-click as they turn. At one spot, the suburban yards give way to one big corporate lawn, I pull the bike over and lie there staring at the sky. Cold, but comfortable. Disconnected. Loose. Stepping away from everything. No expectations to meet. Just lying there.

I'm back on the bike laughing and peddling, peddling, peddling. No one around. No cars. No people. Everything is open, free. I take turn after turn, down streets I don't know. Hours later things begin to look familiar and I come out close to my grandmother's house in the next town. I take a known road. I go back to my parents' garage – the giant two story garage detached from the house. I climb to the upper floor and fall asleep.

I talk to my mother first, after my father has gone off for work. All during the day she calls my father. He agrees that I can stay if I go to see some kind of counselor, a shrink. By now I'm desperate. In Barnes and Noble, I read something about Ayurvedic medicine. In the phone book I find a woman, a psychiatrist, who supposedly knows Ayurvedic treatment. I make an appointment.

Through the waiting room door, I hear some of the conversation with another patient. Problems with jobs and boyfriends. I shake my head as I go in. I don't need counseling, I need a good gut. I tell her about the history of the disease, ask her questions about

 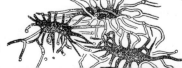

how emotions play a role, about the helpfulness of meditation. She claims to use meditation to help balance out her job of seeing troubled patients. She suggests some Ayurvedic medicine and a change in diet, including consuming dairy products. She professes surprise that I cannot tolerate lactose. She thinks that dairy will help balance my emotional state. I order the Ayurvedic medicine, take it as directed for a couple of weeks, and see no change.

The second visit is the last. She wants to explore childhood memories but I tell her nothing bad has happened other than colitis related experiences. When the appointment ends, she declares me OK.

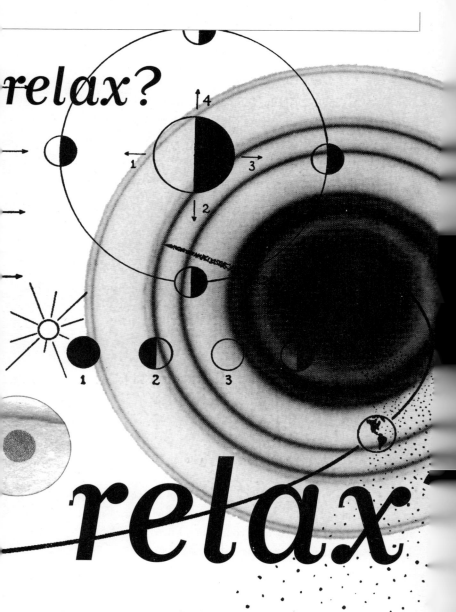

MORE DOCTORS

I'm sitting on a freshly papered examination table at TownCenter Medical. My hip's in continuous pain, my lower back out of joint. Digestion remains terrible. I'm going to the general practitioner one more time to see if he has any suggestions – anything at all which may help the situation. He doesn't have patience.

"Many of my patients have inflammatory bowel disease. You should spend more time relaxing..."

Relax! Relax! I lost 25 pounds in the hospital for the second time! My parents are paying for my medical expenses because I'm not well enough to get a job! I've felt this way for nearly six years and I don't know of any alternatives except surgery or steroids and he tells me to...relax!? He must have caught the frustration on my face as he added, "I find that with my job I also have to spend time unwinding. I enjoy reading Patrick O' Brian. He writes historical novels about sea voyages..."

Relax! Back at home I retreat to the garage. Hoisting up the old Everlast punching bag I feel fear. Strange nostalgia. Six years ago I was in the same place, same garage, same tools hanging on the wall, same stains on the concrete. The past years of college have slipped away, now I'm back. Pieces of tape on the punching bag mark knuckle-sized targets. The blue bag looks dull now, dusty and worn. On the workbench, buried beneath piles of boxes and tools, sits an old cassette player – the one that needed to be duct taped closed. I plug it in and hit play. A single booms out...

"Punching out the suckers and wonderin' how I do it...
They call me D-Nice...
I remain in this mode, very cool, very calm,
There's no sweat in my palm..."

A cassette tape from garage training. The summer before senior year of high school. But without the door open, without the sun in the afternoon, without James, Jon, Sam, and Keith.

Now it's only me. Ghosts haunt the garage. Piles of junk and that

relax? relax? relax

bag hanging there. Not wanting to get stuck in my thoughts
I scrounge around for a heavy pair of work gloves, turn up the
volume, and begin batting away at the bag. No kicks: it feels
like a knife blade in the back to raise my knee.

Afterwards I go inside, put on a sweatshirt over my sweaty t-shirt,
drink some water, and retreat to the inner basement. Lights out.
I place my feet on the desk, close my eyes, and visit the hill.

+   +   +   +

My aunt mails a clipping from a magazine. It's a small news item
about a book called *Food and the Gut Reaction* by Elaine Gottschall,
which details a diet to relieve colitis and Crohn's disease.

Not able to find the book in the local Barnes & Noble, I special
order it from the Yale Coop. When it arrives I flip through it
and notice that half the volume consists of recipes. I don't read a full
explanation of the diet but it includes vegetables, nuts, and even
raw fruit. I haven't touched fruits or nuts in nearly seven years;
some cooked vegetables are OK, but not raw salad.

The final strike against the book comes in the index. I recently
found one thing which improves my gut: acidophilus capsules.
In my mind, part of any diet treatment has to include this
supplement. When I see no mention of acidophilus in the index,
I return the book to the shelf and walk out empty-handed –
to my later regret.

+   +   +   +

Hearing of my situation, my father's boss insists I seek answers from
a doctor who "saved" him by diagnosing a rare disease missed by
other physicians. I'm driving my father's Buick from one suburb to
another, swimming on the front bench seat, pulling myself up by
the steering wheel to look over the dashboard. The car is huge, one
step away from a hearse. There aren't many people out. Everyone's at
work except for the elderly and people who fall through the cracks,
like me. Unemployed, no discernible future. My eyes stay dead
straight. Don't want to look back, don't want to think. I turn into
the driveway for the doctor's office. The sterile manicured lawn,

stifling

swimming in the buick

the industrial carpeted reception. Everything professional, the way you'd expect. Stifling.

The doc's heavy, Sanderson's body type, but he is hope. I hold a sheaf of papers with my medical history: symptoms, hospital stays, prescriptions. Over the past two days I've taken my 1990 history and updated it for 1995. The questions start.

"Where did you go to college?"

I tell him the school.

He looks at me accusingly. "How did you get into that college?! Where did you go to high school?"

"North Haven High." It's the public school in my town, not as good as the one in this doctor's town.

He spends the next five minutes complaining about getting his kids into college. Looking me over, he nods once, he's figured out how I made it.

"You're Iranian? Some kind of Persian?"

"No." Before he starts again, I begin explaining my problem. He cuts me off.

"Whoa!" He holds up his hand. "Stop. You have ulcerative colitis."

"Yes."

"And your doctor was Dr. Brennan?"

"Yes."

"Then why do you need me? His practice knows everything. I can't help you. This ends the appointment."

After no more than sixty seconds of discussing my health situation, I leave with a $100 doctor's bill, and a strong desire to fight. I drive out of the office area, go home, and hole up in the basement.

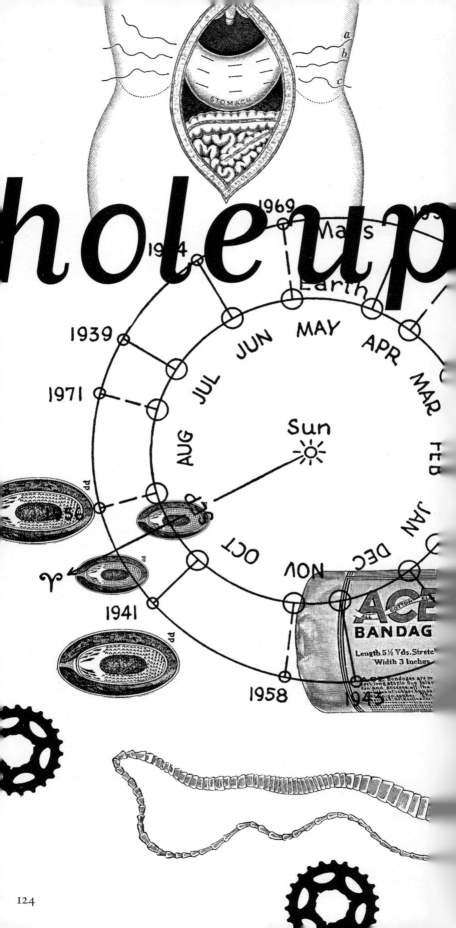

holeup

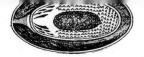

KILLING TIME

It ain't so pretty. High school sports banquet. Down at the Knights of Columbus Hall. The paper tablecloths and good buffet food. The podium and award plaques. Sponsorship by the Tomahawk Club. Everyone wearing their best clothes, mismatched suits and ties. Guys laughing, tearing up the table cloths. The cheap-looking metal chairs cluing you in to the worn tables beneath all that white paper. But the night has energy, it has a feel to it. It's the end of the season, time to relax, recount, laugh. This is part of the ceremony. It comes four months after the week of double and triple sessions, the start of the season where you ran, sweated, and dehydrated, ran some more, threw whatever it was you had into practice, trying to prove yourself so that you could play in the big games. Our team, the soccer team practiced next to the football team during those double-sessions. We would have our morning road runs, our morning practices, our morning sprints which had to be completed in time or they had to be run again and again and again. You'd better be fast or there'd be no water and you'd be cutting into the midday break. Those few hours in between practices where you'd rush home, eat as much as you could and collapse downstairs or go to someone's house with a pool. Either way, you had to focus and make that run. It consisted of 4 sets of 6 runs across the width of the field and back; if you went over the 90 second time limit you had to run it again and again until you made it. The sports-banquet with its large pasta dishes is a world away. People have ace bandages underneath khaki pants. They no longer have to take Tylenol, Advil, and other pain killers to keep their sore, strained muscles active.

Jon Cavallaro, one of the football team captains, comes up to the podium. No one's sure why the team chose Jon, he wasn't that good and he sure didn't have the poise of the previous captain who pulled all A's in advanced courses, was elected class president, and played quarterback. Jon had his speech in hand on a crumpled piece of paper. As he lumbered up to the podium, the cheers started: "Cavallaro!" "Go get 'em, Johnnie!" "Speech! Speech!" The speech went along the lines of "we had a fine season." I expected it to go into the usual: "We played this team, we played that team, remember what happened in the game when..." But Johnny squinted hard at that piece of paper and came up with thank-yous. "I'd like to

memory

get it all out

thank the coaches because they're the best of the best." He said it loud and proud, his voice boomed across Knight of Columbus. In half a year, he'd be working for the town, his future sealed. This might be the last time he held a position of such honor, he loved these people and he was going to tell them so.

"And I'd like to thank the cheerleaders because they're the best of the best." Pause, wait for applause, acknowledgement.

"Go, Cavallaro!"

"And, I'd like thank the parents who raised us, they're the best of the best!"

Old Jon was stumping now, he went through the parents, the fundraisers, the people who kept score, the people who drove the bus to away games, the guy who kept the equipment in order, the water boys. He was driving himself toward tears, everyone else to exasperation. When would this end? And then he brought it to a close:

"Finally, I'd like to thank the players, because without them there would be no team. Thank you."

"Yeah, Cavallaro!" "No one could argue with those words!"

My feelings were cocky then, comparing my future to Cavallaro's. Hell, now I practically envy Cavallaro, I see him hanging out by the gas station once in a while. Sometimes I imagine my own banquet. I'm recovered, I'm walking to the podium with my crumpled list, going up there to say thanks to those who got me throug There's some family, a couple of friends. Recently there's only my mom whose hair is turning white with worry and who tries to cook up dishes which will put weight back on my bones. There's my mom and there's Axl Rose. He doesn't say anything, he's more of a shadow. Sitting with the band, their tablecloth tattered up, throwing wads of paper at each other. I just want to thank them for showing me a way to help wrench this whole disease right out of my system. Each day, around mid-morning, the house is empty. It's me with no place to go. Not a fan of daytime TV, and in no mood to read, just pacing, around. Axl goes into the stereo.

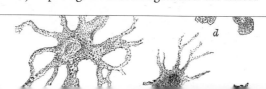

There are these mini-speakers in the ceiling which can shake the room. My mom listens only to classical. My dad never listens to music. But I let this thing reach its potential. Put in the disk, skip ahead to the 12 minute long song *Coma*, and turn up the volume. I stand in the dining room with those speakers pointed down at my head, screaming along at the top of my lungs. Stomping around, shaking, screaming. "YOU CAUGHT ME IN A COMA AND I DON'T THINK I WANNA ...EVER COME BACK TO THIS...WORLD AGAIN...SUSPENDED DEEP IN A SEA OF BLACK..."

I scream till my vocal cords strain. I want to rip out whatever's in my body, get it out, get it all out. I'm screaming for my life, shouting for my life. Everyone I know, everything I know has moved on again. I'm sitting watching it, going nowhere. Picture riding my bike. The woman from the end of my junior year, who by default I'm now in love with the image of. Faces flashing by of people from 8th grade through college. Where the hell is everyone? Where am I? What have I done to myself? I have to tear away, clear myself out. The CD stops, I'm wrung out, near tears. I get that mixed up feeling, that last 100 meter sprint feeling. *Coma*'s the last track on the CD. When the silence hits, I slowly walk over to the machine and restart the song. I'm gonna get it all out of me, here and now. I'm going to walk out into the sunset. Rediscover my life, get back on whatever path...

By the time the song ends a second time, I open the door and step outside. I'm barefoot, wearing sweat pants and no shirt. Its cold, the rain's coming down. I just stand there, I glance down and see my heart going, rib cage expanding and deflating. I stare at the clouds. After a while, my feet become as cold as the bricks. I walk back, shivering as I close the door. Just another day. Yeah. Yeah.

Thank you Guns-n-Roses, because without you, there would be no music to scream to. Without music, there would be oblivion.

rip it out
ip it out

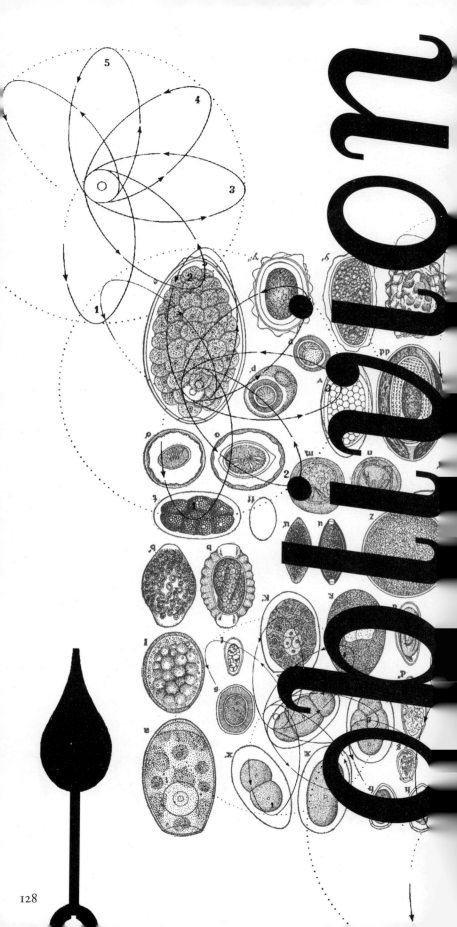

JOB?

My father's a damn persistent guy. Six weeks after the declining of the Big Consulting Company interview, breaking the wall, and being declared clean by the shrink without ever having to go Freudian, I listen while he eases me into another of his plans.

"There's another guy whose company does consulting. I spoke to him after a meeting yesterday. We're on the economic development committee together. I showed him your resume–"

"What do they do?" I'm confused.

"Same thing as the other company, computer consulting. But they're a local company, all of their work is around here. I showed him your resume, he turned it over and went right to the computer section."

In the computer section I don't have much listed. The only class that comes close is a Lotus 1-2-3 course worth half the usual credits. The final project became a bit complex but it definitely wasn't programming.

"Lombardi said that if you'd like, he could set up an interview. It's up to you. No pressure."

I agree. If I stay in the house, I'll drive everyone crazy, including myself.

The morning of the interview I go to the gym. In between sets, dizzy and sweating, I psych myself up with the idea that a half hour exchange of words can get me money, health benefits, and out of the house! I own a pair of suit pants bought at a going out of business sale and also a white shirt. I borrow a tie from my dad's closet, bring along a folder containing a pad and extra copies of my resume, and head out. The interviewer is on-site at a job and I meet her in the building cafeteria. I've been out of it so long that her appearance surprises me. She's my age but her suit and hairstyle give me the impression of experience, someone who has already spent years in the real world. I feel a bit foolish, knowing my dad knows her boss. But it doesn't matter, my focus snaps on.

what do they do?

After introductions, she asks standard questions about my educational background and what I have been doing. I piece together a somewhat coherent story based on graduating, going into the post-bac program, having a change of heart, and now I am here. I omit mention of hospitals, vomiting, and shitting blood. After all, it's been at least two hours since I last saw any blood in the bowl.

I am going to compensate for my lack of work history with words. I want to show that I embody the work ethic and never-say-die spirit. I want to invoke David Sarnoff, the man who grew up in Hell's Kitchen, and supported his entire family selling newspapers, the first step in tirelessly building a business, eventually bringing the country AM radio, FM radio, television. Horatio Alger. But before I invoke these images, she starts off with the computer questions:

"Are you experienced with procedural programming?"

"Not exactly."

"Tell me what you think of client-server programming?"

I looked at some computer books at Barnes and Noble the days before and manage a general description.

"Do you have experience with relational database design?"

(I won't lie to you, but I used to be the best). "Most of my experience was with..."

In the beginning of the interview, she smiles, but during the computer questions, she goes flat. Boy, I sound bad.

I go home happy that I have gotten through the interview and that my clothes have held together – I still use a modified belt with an extra hole.

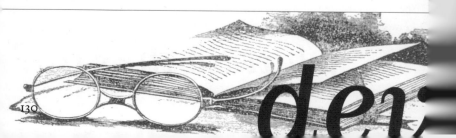

PROGRAMMING

The next afternoon, on the phone, I receive a report from Lombardi.

"She liked you. The interview went well. But she didn't feel you had enough experience. But if you could find a Cobol class, I'll bring you in to try some work at our development center." From the papers handed out by my interviewer, I learned that this is a place at the company's main office where they bring contract work in-house. I thank him and hit the yellow pages.

Southern Connecticut State University, The University of New Haven, Quinnipiac College, UCONN, Albertus Magnus, Central, Sacred Heart, Fairfield, Yale, Wesleyan, Eastern Connecticut...In the next hour I call a dozen universities which offer summer courses. None of them offer Cobol.

Still caught up in the possibility of work, I drive to Quinnipiac, a local college.

Luckily, the professor who teaches the Cobol class is in his office. I talk to him about the possibility of taking a private class.

"It is a very difficult subject. You can't simply rush and learn it. You need to take a semester-long course."

I tell him the situation, the possibility of work contingent on taking a class, tell him my mom has taught there part-time for twenty years.

"As I said, it's not something that you just go and do."

I change my tactics, asking for names of other people, then for guidance, an old syllabus.

No. No. No. He impatiently declines. In the end I request the name of a text book – somewhere to start. No.

I leave frustrated.

The last possibility of taking a class is a text-based self-tutorial on the mainframe at my father's workplace. The consulting head agrees that this will be enough to give me a trial internship at the company's development center. For a week I go to my father's workplace for 2–3 hours a day. He has a friend, Harold, placed in a side office off a major hallway. It's a tucked-away space, unnoticed in the building complex which holds over 3,000 workers. Harold's area has an unused back room with two terminals. I have access to one of them. No mouse, only a keyboard and monochrome green monitor wired into the mainframe. A computer instructor from the workplace has set up the account in my father's name. I sit reading screens about the Cobol language and working my way through multiple choice questions. The instructor also brings along a teacher's copy of an old Cobol book. This becomes my main learning material. I trade the monochrome screen for sitting back home in the basement with the Cobol book and a legal pad. With no computer, I write the programs down on the pad. This allows me to learn the language.

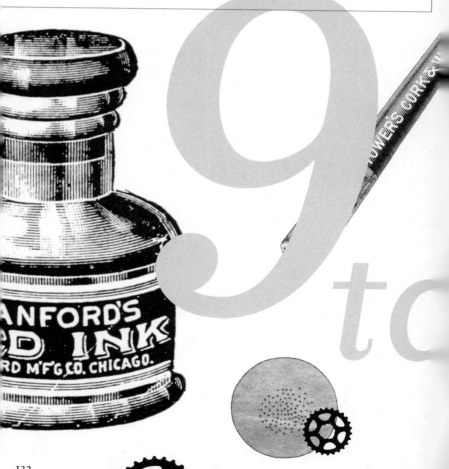

WORKING

Although I still cannot survive intense work hours, this company is OK, 9 to 5. For the development center trial, I wear a jacket and tie. The lost weight from last summer never returned. I no longer have gluteus muscles nor much of a waist. The company headquarters is thirty minutes away. When I cross the parking lot to the building entrance, I keep a hand discreetly by my side, holding up my pants.

In the first days of my internship, the transition from yellow legal pad to keyboard goes slowly. There is another language, called Job Control Language (JCL), which is needed for Cobol to interact with files. It resembles 1,000 license plate numbers jumbled onto the screen. At the end of the day I leave exhausted, the stomach in its usual post-lunch bloated mode. But it's good to be around people. Most of the company's employees are fulltime and work onsite at various client offices. The development center often has one person "on the bench," or between assignments. But it also has a half dozen working mothers who are able to arrange their schedules more easily because they work in-house. Two of the women, Sandra and Robin take me in, helping me get started, helping take away the feeling that I have somehow snuck in this place undeserved. My first project goes well and they send me into the field.

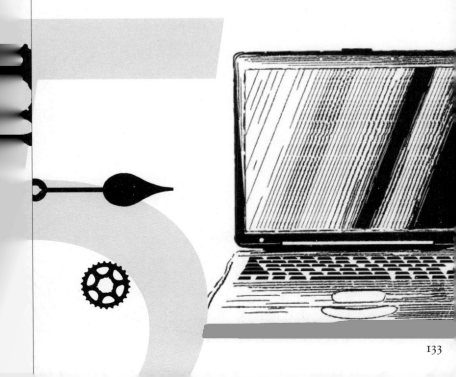

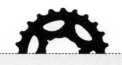

date:
10/8/95

days since diagnosed:
2,121

age:
23

weight:
145

location:
cubicle, middletown, ct

medication:
*azulfidine supplement, multi-vitamin,
acidophilus capsule, aloe vera juice*

general symptoms:
*frequent b.m.'s (unformed or running);
bloated stomach after eating;
occasional blood in stool; "brain fog";
back/hip pain*

diet restrictions:
*no dairy, no raw fruits or vegetables,
no nuts*

attitude:
try not to think about it

GIRLFRIEND

In February of 1996, my health stays on the borderline. I do some
stretches, some mild weight lifting, walk out of work stiff-backed
and exhausted, and generally feel like half a person. The programming continues to go well but I still find myself visiting back-up
loos within the office building.

Two friends from high school are back in town and we begin to
hang out together. Often this means meeting up and playing foosball in my parents' basement. Sam is taking classes and working in
a lab in order to beef up a med school application and Frank has
returned from a year-long backpacking trip across Australia and the
Middle East. He temps in an office and works at a coffee shop in
order to pay off his loans.

On one weekend, we go to a birthday party thrown for Sam's sister,
Sumi, who is a year older. The party is thrown by her "successful"
friends. Talking to them and hearing about their careers leave us
depressed. The party is held in an apartment with a thick carpet
and a cat. I'm allergic to cats and succumb to sniffling and watery
eyes. We soon fall back to sitting on a couch, telling jokes, and waiting for the food. At one point, with the music playing and everyone
engaged in conversation, the doorbell rings. I'm near the bell, the
only one to hear it. When I open the door, a cute woman stands
on the steps. My eyes linger for a second but then I notice the six
foot guy behind her and his friend. I say hi, let them in and return
to my corner. Sumi, Sam's sister later introduces her as N.. For the
rest of the afternoon, I glance in her direction, but we don't talk.

The next day, in a burst of bravery, I call Sumi and ask for the
woman's number. I hastily scrawl it on the back of a road atlas.
I retire to the basement, sit cross-legged on the floor with the
phone in front of me, take a few slow breaths, and call. She seems
distracted, aloof. We talk for about ten minutes. She's a graduate
student in graphic design. Somehow, by the time I hang up, I have
a date for the following Friday.

We go to a seafood restaurant in New Haven, dimly lit, table near
the water. She suggests going to a bar afterwards. I have another
drink, a beer. The date ends near midnight. Walking home, across

the street, I decide to hold her hand. I won't even attempt a kiss, just take her hand. It's not a straight forward motion. Her left hand is thrust into the pocket of a bulky winter coat. The sides of the coat don't touch her body, so I think that reaching into the pocket to take her hand will be OK. We are already walking so close together anyway.

I reach for her hand. She resists, pulling away. My hand becomes trapped in the pocket. We are in the middle of the street, my arm seemingly stretched six feet as I struggle to get my hand out.

"What are you doing?!"

"I wasn't doing anything, just trying to hold your hand." I retreat, my hands at shoulder level, palms facing her in surrender position. "Really, I wasn't even trying to kiss you. I just wanted to hold your hand."

We cross the street and end up at the steps of her building. She stands on the first step looking down while I remain on the sidewalk. She's yelling.

"...I'm not afraid of you!"

She glares at me from the steps. I lower my eyes, confused. I catch sight of a keychain in her hands. All of her keys are attached to a tattered plastic doll.

"That's the ugliest thing I've ever seen."

"What do you mean?"

"Your key chain. It's horrible."

She glares.

"Good night."

"Bye." She turns and heads up the stairs. As I open my car door, I imagine that before I can get home, she will tell Sumi about her awful date, Sumi will call Sam, and I'll be the target of laughter at

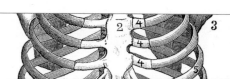

the next foosball game. I cannot understand it: I thought we got along so well at dinner.

The following night there is a party thrown by someone at Sam's lab. N. and Sumi plan on being there. After the previous night, I have no desire to go. In addition, the alcohol has thrown my system off and I spend the day feeling washed out, pale, and making multiple trips to the loo.

+   +   +

A couple of days after the initial encounter I receive a call from Sumi.

"Why don't you call N.?"

"Call N.? Did she tell you how the evening went? I had a great time in the beginning but at the end it —"

"Well, I know that she wants you to call her."

"Really?"

"Yes."

For our second date we see an Indian movie, *The Bandit Queen*. It's a nonfiction story about a woman who is married off as a child bride to an old man. She runs away from him, runs away from her family, and joins a gang of bandits who rob rural villages. At one point she is caught and raped by nearly all the men in one of the villages. Later, her gang massacres these men. If any movie has the potential to suck away romance, this is it. But we meet again the following morning. For a project, she wants to photograph some areas in Bridgeport, Connecticut, one of the most blighted cities in the country. Despite the hand-holding episode, *The Bandit Queen*, and romantic trips to burned-out houses, we continue to see each other.

My routine becomes go to work, visit N., talk on the phone with N. I keep a daily planner which includes a section on hours of sleep.

For days it reads: 2 hours, 3 hours, 1 hour. I live on adrenaline; my body isn't falling apart; the energy of the relationship sparks me on.

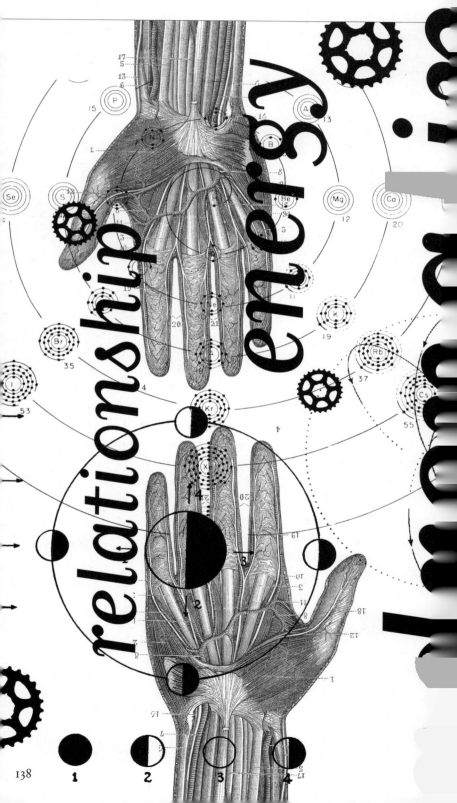

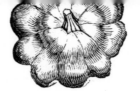

NO MEAT

That summer I move to New Haven. My health remains the same,
I simply pay less attention to it. A woman on my project team at
work is a vegetarian – a fact that always comes up when the team
has pizza parties. I talk to her and find that she follows a strict diet
after having stomach ulcers years before. After that conversation
and more reading, I decide to become a vegetarian for a month.
In a vegetarian grocery in New Haven, I find aisles of products new
to me, including Rice Dream – milk made with rice! This means
a chance to have cereal again! Between rice dream, a rice cooker,
and tofu, my diet becomes quite "light." But I don't feel any
significant effect, definitely not better. After the month, I return
to eating meat.

+   +   +   +

I spot a flier for free yoga classes stapled to a light post. I scribble
down the address on the back of an ATM receipt. The classes are
held in a former factory about a mile from my apartment. The
ceilings are 20 feet high and a refinished hardwood floor stretches
across a giant square room. People line the perimeter, their backs
to the wall. We start off sitting with the bottoms of our feet pressed
together, a regular stretch for the inner thighs. The instructor,
a tall, energetic woman in her mid-50s leads the class, guiding
everyone on how to breath, feeling the breath going in, letting the
floating ribs fall as we breathe out. After several minutes we move
to another pose and then another, always concentrating on breathing. In a standing pose, she takes a look at my flat feet and orders
me to raise my arches, saying that over time, my feet won't be
pancaking out. The class lasts 90 minutes and afterwards I feel
pain free! No aches in the hip, no aches in the shoulders, I feel
close to springy, bouncing. When I see N. I can barely contain
my excitement – the class is amazing.

On Saturday morning, with the free classes still in effect, I take
N. back with me. But when I enter the room, things appear
differently. Instead of sitting along the perimeter, people sit in
orderly rows, facing a different instructor. She's much younger
and barks out orders like an 8th grade gym teacher. There's no

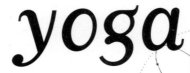

pleasant voice, no talk about breathing. Instead the female version of Mr. Scarpolini, the junior high gym teacher, has arrived. In those junior high years, one game we played with Mr. Scarpolini was with a giant earth ball.

"Gentleman, the ball is an island. Everyone wants to be on the island. Get on the island any way you can. But no punching."

And the whistle blew. It was a great game. But that is a different time – this is a yoga class to stretch and loosen the body, not tame a bunch of sugar-fueled, hormone-laden junior high kids. Leaving the class I feel stretched but not peaceful. N. says it isn't as good as her aerobics class. She cannot stand the yoga woman's grating voice.

I find out the teaching times of the original instructor and attend more classes. After one session, I can place my foot back on the highest rungs of the stepladder, without any back pain. My spine is getting re-aligned or something – things are falling into place. I haven't been able to do that stretch without a pull in my back for at least three years.

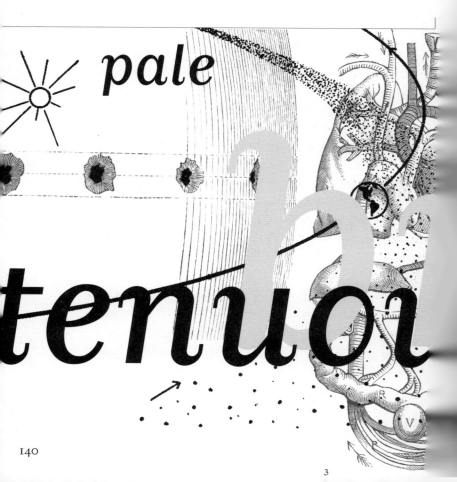

pale

tenuo

TOO FAST

I sit in the second cubicle on a row named Easy Street. Vaulted ceilings loom forty feet above the hundreds of IT personnel cubicles. The hermetically sealed, tinted windows dim the floor, leaving everyone dependent on fluorescent lights. Each morning I make my way up the steps, across the floor, and into the cubicle. I flip on my machines, enter my passwords, and work. Or, during lulls, I spin my chair so my back faces passersby, open a folder of documentation, and read a novel tucked inside.

Leaving the office I feel stiffer and a more drained than the day before.

With yoga and various supplement experiments, from acidophilus to aloe vera, I start feeling better – my stomach still bloats up but I don't see blood in the toilet bowl.

The fragile boost in health along with being around N. and her classmates motivates me to get on with my life. If this is the way it is going to be, so be it. My job is increasingly redundant. I've taken some company run software training classes but it seems doubtful that I'll be able to use the skills – the company has too much work for the looming Year 2000 date change "crisis." I find out that a college in upstate New York runs a satellite school in Hartford, Connecticut. Started decades ago to help ease an engineering shortage, the school offers degrees for working people in computer science, engineering, and management.

I sign up for two prerequisite computer science classes in the fall semester. Beginning in September, I trade my once-a-week yoga class and stretching after work for two 3-hour-long night classes, each with an accompanying 90 minutes of driving. I approach the classes in a disciplined manner – re-copying all my notes within 24 hours of lecture and keeping up with homework. By October, the extra sitting and lack of exercise break my tenuous grip on health. My complexion becomes pale and washed out, my back aches all the time, and the gut goes bad: diarrhea, increased bloating, blood, the works.

washed out

BAD ORGANS

In November 1996, the right upper abdominal area near my liver begins hurting. At first I think I've pulled a muscle. For the next two days I slump over my desk in the cubicle trying to prop myself up on my elbows so it will look as if I'm reading.

The inability to keep liquids or food down begins again and I call my new doctor, Dr. Lee. I switched to him after the last hospital visit, two years before. Dr. Lee checks me into the hospital where a colonoscopy viewed through a blazing color monitor shows full blown ulcerative colitis throughout the large intestine. I check out of the hospital with a strong prednisone prescription.

A follow up appointment at Dr. Lee's office takes on a serious tone. Months before, during my first appointments I told him that I didn't want to take any medication and filled him in on my use of acidophilus, aloe vera, and the avoidance of dairy and corn syrup. He was supportive, reminding me that the medicine was there. He said that so many of his patients suffered despite the medications that he was interested in how I fared with my "experiments." Now, after a trip to the hospital and the colonoscopy, he conveys the seriousness of my situation:

"Your intestine looks like bloody hamburger. Also your liver enzyme counts are extremely high. Close to the profile of an alcoholic. I had blood samples drawn to check your serum alkaline phosphatase level. These levels are also extremely high."

"What does that mean?"

"The levels shown by the blood tests indicate primary schlerosing cholangitis–a rare liver disease. It's rare in that not many people have it. However, most people who do have it also have a condition such as ulcerative colitis. I had the blood samples drawn twice to confirm the counts. It's a serious matter."

He went on to explain that there's no effective treatment except for a liver transplant.

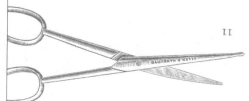

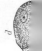

"I want to confirm the schlerosing cholangitis by doing a liver biopsy. It's an outpatient procedure. Also, for the ulcerative colitis, you may want to consider surgery."

Still spinning from the hospital stay, this news throws me off balance. My colon and now my liver – two major organs in serious trouble.

When I was in the hospital, N. came each day. Her face at the hospital haunts me. I never want someone to be so sad on my account. Also, I cannot handle the idea of quitting another academic semester. I feel crushed, being pulled inexorably down into the abyss: surgery seems the only solution for the colitis, my liver is having serious problems, I have had another hospital stay, I have abandoned my apartment after fewer than six months and I'm convalescing at my parents' house. I'm screwed once again, quitting everything.

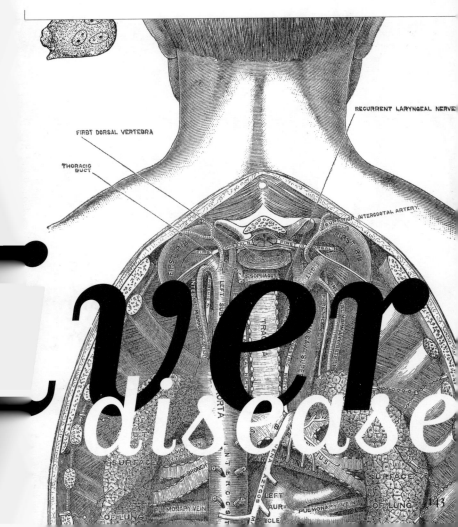

BACK ON PREDNISONE

But it doesn't happen that way. With the prednisone screaming through my body I return to work missing only three days. I lose weight again. My pants don't fit so I wear two pairs of boxers and re-notch my belt as an alternative to getting a new one.

I miss only a week of classes and with the drugs keeping the wheels turning, dizzy and propped up on prednisone, I return to finish the semester. I bring a curl bar with light weights on it back to the apartment. I press and curl near collapse, a madman in a small studio apartment.

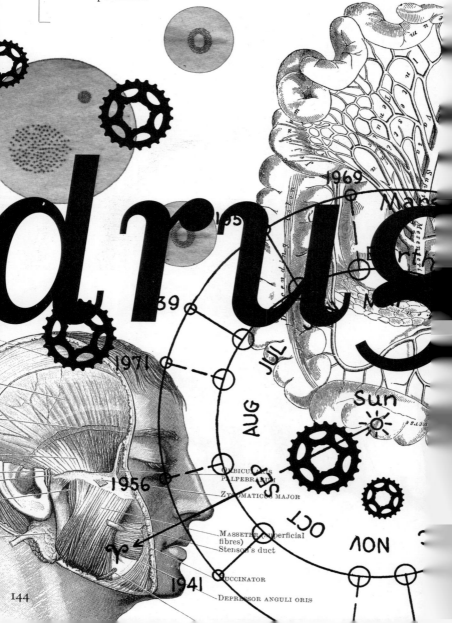

date:
12/10/1996

days since diagnosed:
2,543

age:
24

weight:
140

location:
new haven, ct

medication:
prednisone, azulfidine supplement,
multi-vitamin, acidophilus capsule,
aloe vera juice

general symptoms:
severe ulcerative colitis;
schlerosing cholangitis

diet restrictions:
no dairy, no raw fruits or vegetables,
no nuts

attitude:
hopeful

1946

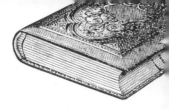

ANOTHER HOPE

I don't want to be in the hospital again. Period. Before my classes end, I accompany N. to the art library where she needs to complete research. I bring a math book, a yellow legal pad, and a lead pencil to knock out a problem set. It's the winter of 1996 and my work-place remains primitive in regard to internet access – my computer still doesn't have a mouse. However, in the library sit two new machines with 21 inch monitors and a super-fast university connec-tion. I search for ulcerative colitis and come across a book titled *Breaking the Vicious Cycle*. It's available for purchase and claims to alleviate colitis and Crohn's disease through diet. The website doesn't offer much information, but I risk the $20.

When the book arrives in the mail I read it through twice. The author, Elaine Gottschall, focuses on the inability of inflammatory bowel disease (IBD) patients to digest certain carbohydrates. She describes a "vicious cycle" where injury to the surface of the small intestine leads to the inability to properly digest the carbohydrates in many foods including bread, pasta, rice, and milk. When the body cannot properly digest these foods, the undigested carbohy-drates become energy which fuels bacterial overgrowth in the intestinal tract. The small intestine becomes injured further and responds to the increase of bacterial by-products by creating more mucus. In turn, the mucus leads to further impaired digestion and the cycle escalates, resulting in symptoms such as diarrhea and eventually ulcerative colitis and Crohn's disease. The source of the original injury may start with bacterial overgrowth in the small intestine due to reasons such as interference with the high acidity of the stomach due to overuse of antacids or age, malnutrition or poor diet, and antibiotics.

The studies cited in the book include a description of a well-studied synthetic Elemental Diet, usually administered through a stomach tube, that has proved successful in alleviating intestinal disorders including Crohn's disease. The Elemental Diet is prohibitive because of cost and when it is stopped, symptoms gradually return. However, the main carbohydrate in the Elemental Diet is glucose which the stomach does not need to break down – it is simply absorbed. Based on this and other studies, the author proposes

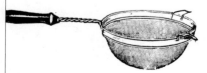

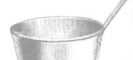

a diet which contains no carbohydrates other than those found in specific vegetables, meats and fish, fruits, honey, nuts, yogurt (which has been fermented at least 24 hours to break down all of the lactose), and harder cheeses. In other words, the diet avoids carbohydrates an injured intestine cannot break down, including pasta, bread, rice, and soy. The diet also avoids all processed foods and added sugars. The underlying idea is to eat what the body can digest. It is known as the Specific Carbohydrate Diet (SCD).

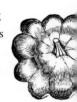

Studies and explanations fill the first forty-two pages of the book, followed by the diet. With my body in shambles, it sounds too good. If I weren't so desperate, I'm not sure I would try it, but I decide to give it a shot. Not a meek, half-hearted try. The author writes in boldface that the diet will work only with **determined adherence**. No problem. I open the cupboards and begin throwing most of my food into the garbage: boxes of rice dream, pasta, aloe vera juice, a loaf of bread, packaged foods with any type of sugar or preservative. After the emptying of the cupboards comes a trip to the supermarket.

With muzak playing in the background I keep to the perimeter of the store: vegetables, meat, butter, cheddar cheese, milk to make yogurt, some apples and ripe bananas, and a successful search for dry curd cottage cheese – also known as farmer's cheese.

On the prednisone I can eat anything and not feel pain, but I also feel numb and confused on the drug. My brain turns into a high speed record, and in between work and school projects I don't see any definite outward changes except that I spend a lot of time cooking for this new diet. But there is a change. After six weeks on the diet a follow up blood test for my liver shows that the serum alkaline phosphatase levels, indicative of schlerosing cholangitis, have returned to normal. My liver biopsy is put on hold – permanently.

In March and April I stop the prednisone and slowly build my strength back up. My father purchases another house to renovate and I begin helping out at night – my body struggling with the work after a day in the cubicle but feeling better for it.

I continue to follow the diet, buying a food processor to assist my

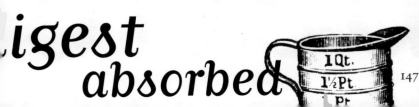

cooking. Grain is not allowed on the diet, but breads may be made using almond flour. I join an e-mail list for the diet and read the posts each day. The encouragement and tips from veterans and stories of newcomers continue to motivate me. I feel we are a rag-tag team navigating out of a nightmare. A guy on the diet in Denmark even puts up a website – a relatively new phenomenon in 1997. One person has found a source of almond flour in California – a wholesale company that ships twenty-five pound boxes to individuals. I order my first box, find the consistency much finer than what I can make with the food processor, and go into "cake" and "bread" production.

I still feel tired, which I attribute to my adrenals needing to "warm up" again after my last bout of prednisone, but something is missing. The gnawing pain is gone as well as the urgency to use the loo – I achieve solid BM's on a daily basis! I don't feel like I am 17, but I feel better than at ages 18, 19, 20, 21, 22, 23, and 24.

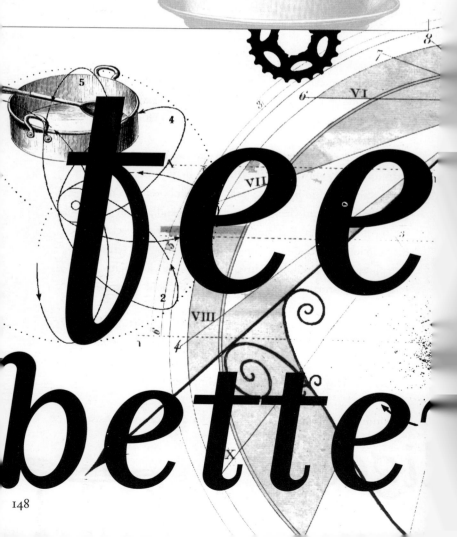

feel
better

GETTING STRONGER

During the summer I take a short, five week computer class.
It passes by quickly and in good health. I gain some weight back
and continue the diet.

Seeing my health improve leaves me confused. I want to revert
to my old thinking – gain all my weight back, sign up for the
gym, go back to karate, run and jump in the streets. But the yoga
suits me for now and N. plans to move to New York City and
work after her final year. I want to move with her but I don't want
to be stuck working on a Year 2000 project. Still hesitant after taking two classes the previous year and landing in the hospital, I sign
up for the final computer prerequisite course in the fall of 1998.

+ *deep breath*

That winter N. and I drive up to Massachusetts, spending a long
weekend together while staying in bed and breakfasts. At a room
in Newburyport, I cannot sleep. After lying there with eyes open
for half an hour, I stand up, take out my notebook and sit on the
two steps leading down to the bathroom. Turning on a dim light, I
make a plan for going back to school at night so that I can join N.
in New York. The school in Hartford offers three full
semesters per year. I scribble down a schedule that will allow me
to finish the 29 credits I need over the next 12 months.

I will have to take out a loan to cover tuition and for the first eight
months I have to work and go to school. But after the first two
semesters, I plan on stopping work. The biggest question mark
is health. Taking a full load of classes and spending 7.30 a.m. to
9.30 p.m. sitting in front of either a computer screen, a windshield
or a lecture won't help out the back or the gut. I decide to buy
a used indoor rowing machine and force myself to get on it after
class. It won't be so bad I think. That night I sit for an hour with
a course book figuring out the credits, the money, everything.
At the end I take a deep breath and return to sleep.

plan

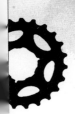

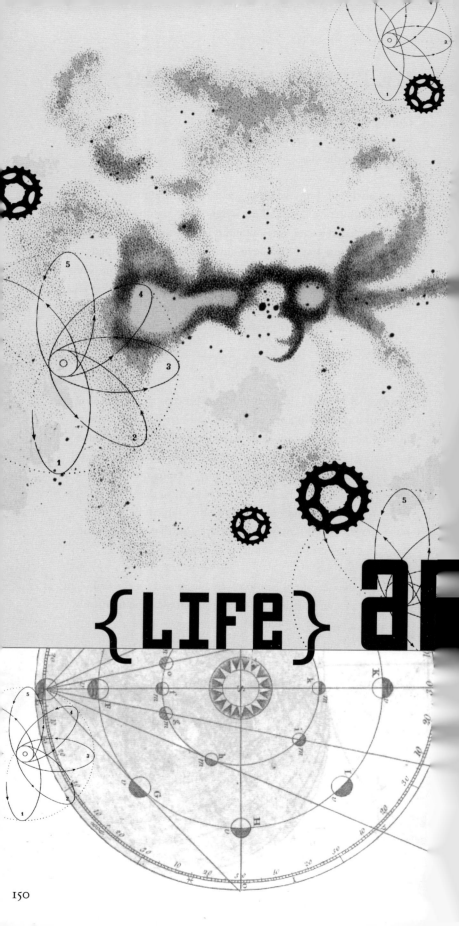

{LIFE} af

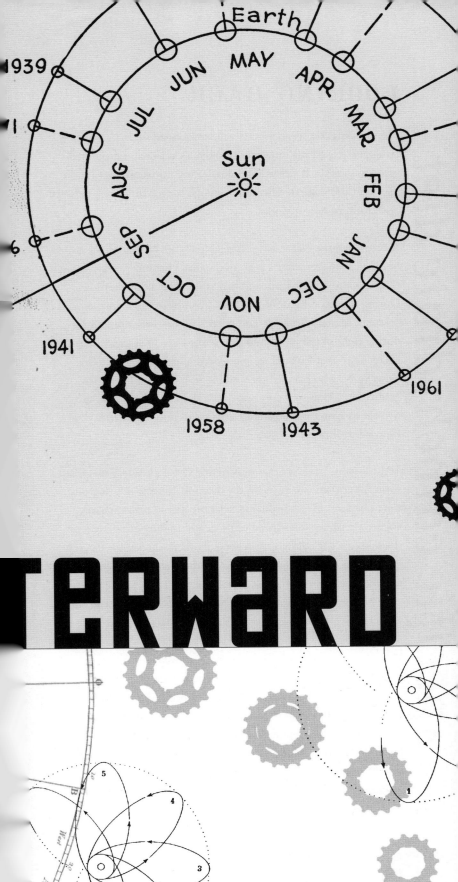

TERWARD

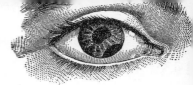

LOOKING BACK

Next week (2009) twenty years will have passed since a gastroen-terologist viewed my intestines through a camera and diagnosed ulcerative colitis. It will also be close to my thirteenth year on the Specific Carbohydrate Diet, long enough for me to make a personal assessment of how it works.

Before using the diet, taking classes after work landed me in the hospital. However, after a year on the diet I became healthy enough to go back to school again and had tapered off all medications. During my second year on the diet, I completed 29 credits of a 30-credit master's degree in computer science – working full-time during eight of the twelve months. I won't say I felt excessively energetic or that I would recommend doing it (I wanted to live closer to N. who planned on working in New York City after graduation). However, even with little sleep, I did not have ulcera-tive colitis symptoms during this period of time. After that year, I moved to Brooklyn.

To be honest, I can say that moving to New York scared me. I had spent fewer than two years on the diet and "intact." During this time I had set up a schedule to keep my diet in place: making yogurt, preparing food ahead of time, and finding a store where I could buy dry curd cottage cheese (farmer's cheese) for making breads with almond flour. Also, before the diet, I had been hospi-talized three times and found it reassuring to have family living close by. Plus, I was moving New York, a place known for its long work hours – not necessarily conducive to a balanced life.

However, my fears soon faded. N. and I moved to a Brooklyn neighborhood where all the food I needed could be purchased with-in a two-block radius. Restaurants accommodated me ("May I have that without the potatoes and with extra vegetables?") My job with a start-up company meant working hard in the summer of 1999 (read: every day in June and three days off in July – two Sundays and a Saturday). However, I usually brought my own lunch to work and for the times I didn't I found a deli with SCD compatible food (they roasted a turkey every day as well as having a good salad

control over my health

bar). I also made sure to stretch in the morning and walk during the day.

The greatest thing I gained was control over my health. From 1989 to 1996 – for over seven years – I could not predict how I would feel from one day to the next. I was living day-to-day but in a miserable way. I couldn't plan ahead with any confidence and the uncertainty wore me down. Now, with a good gut, my life has changed for the better.

fear faded

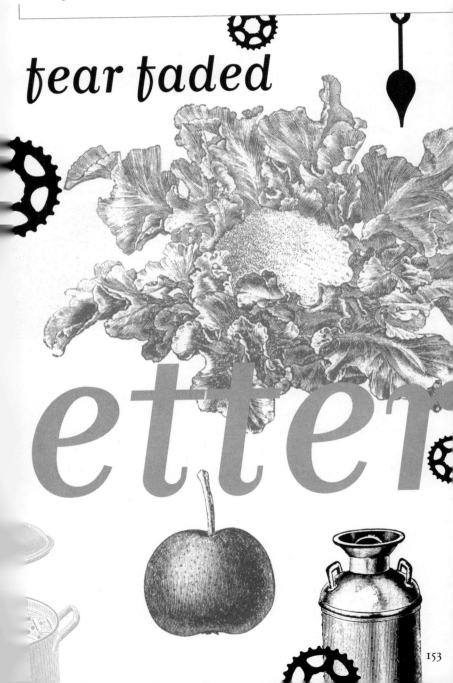

etter

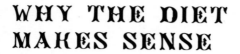

WHY THE DIET MAKES SENSE

Despite *Breaking the Vicious Cycle* selling millions of copies; despite more than twenty websites put up in seven different languages by people successfully using the diet – people spending valuable personal time to inform others; and despite the continued good results people write about on the e-mail list, it's still not the norm for a gastroenterologist to recommend the Specific Carbohydrate Diet. The situation used to confuse me. If something works for so many people and doesn't have any side effects, why don't doctors present it as an option to Inflammatory Bowel Disease (IBD) patients? Some patients might choose an ostomy bag over giving up fast food, but many others would choose the diet. It would improve patients' lives, decrease the money spent on IBD-related medical expenses, and make everyone feel better... well, almost everyone. Pharmaceutical companies who make hundreds of millions of dollars[1] a year selling IBD drugs might not be happy about a diet cutting into their revenue streams (Baker; Barrett).

In addition, although many doctors and the Crohn's & Colitis Foundation of America know of the diet and have heard stories of its success, they say it cannot be advocated, or even discussed, because of lack of studies. However, funding for studies doesn't seem to be coming any time soon. A sentence in a November 11, 2002, Wall Street Journal article on the Specific Carbohydrate Diet summarizes why:

> The failure of the Specific Carbohydrate Diet to gain widespread acceptance within the medical community is a lesson in the grim financial reality of medical research. Doctors don't accept treatments that aren't validated by controlled studies, and drug companies, which fund most medical research, pay to study pills, not diets. (Fiondella R6)

However, even without controlled diet studies, the knowledge of the efficacy of the SCD diet is spreading. The Wall Street Journal article cites an example:

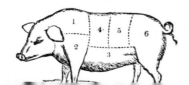

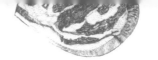

Stuart Ditchek, a New York University associate professor of pediatrics who treats about 25 IBD patients, says that in his experience, 85% of his patients who strictly followed the diet improved. He says many doubting doctors are starting to come around to the idea of the diet, and are now at least willing to consider it. "What you find now is that some doctors will say... 'I'm not sure if it works but you can try it,'" says Dr. Ditchek. "To me that's a victory." (Fiondella R11)

Because of the improved quality of life, I think everyone with IBD should try the diet. However, for those who are "efficiency-minded" with lots to do and for whom popping pills seems preferable to spending valuable time making homemade yogurt, please consider the following:

1. Long term health
With all current IBD medications, the disease is still active: it is only being fought back on a daily basis, causing additional stress to your body. I could scare you by listing the severe side effects of popular IBD medications, but will only mention some of the common ones:

Sulfasalazine (Azulfidine):
"anorexia, headache, nausea, vomiting, gastric distress, and apparently reversible ogliospermia [decreased sperm count]" (Medical Economics Staff 2775)

Mesalamine (Pentasa/Rowasa/Asacol):
"diarrhea, headache, nausea, abdominal pain, dyspepsia, vomiting, rash" (Medical Economics Staff 3240)

Infliximab (Remicade):
"Upper respiratory infection, nausea, abdominal pain, vomiting, headache, pain." (WebMD Inc. "Infliximab")

However, before these more common side effects, the Physicians' Desk Reference contains a capitalized, boldfaced warning similar to the following one:

Serious, even fatal, infections have been reported to occur during

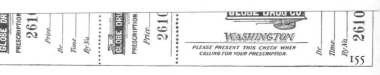

treatment with infliximab. Contact your doctor immediately if you develop signs of infection such as fever or chills; sore throat, coughing, congestion or other signs of infection; redness, pain, or swelling of a skin wound; or burning or difficult urination. (WebMD Inc. "Infliximab")

diet

Corticosteroids (prednisone): insomnia; nausea, vomiting, or stomach upset; fatigue or dizziness; muscle weakness or joint pain; problems with diabetes control; increased hunger or thirst. (WebMD Inc. "Prednisone")

Even with medication, many IBD sufferers describe themselves as living on the borderline. An ulcerative colitis sufferer once described it to me as follows: "I'm never completely sick [bedridden] but I'm never well either."

Despite sticking with their prescriptions, 66% to 75% of people with Crohn's disease will have surgery. Surgery does not mean a cure: 50% of people who undergo operations will require additional surgeries in the future (Zonderman 74). For ulcerative colitis sufferers, 25% to 40% will require surgery (Crohn's & Colitis Foundation of America [CCFA] *Crohn's...Surgery* 9). Despite surgery and medication, the risk of colon cancer increases after having IBD for 8 to 10 years (CCFA *Crohn's...Surgery* 5).

With the diet, the disease is in remission because you eat food which your digestive system can handle. Therefore, the stress of active disease is removed and you no longer have to experience pain, bloating, diarrhea, or blood in the stool. Consequently, you do not have to contend with medications and related side effects, or think about the statistics mentioned above. When you're not feeling well, those statistics become ominous. If you're serious about your long term health, the diet makes sense.

2. Wise use of time

Your diet start-up costs will include extra time in the kitchen, more time reading labels, and educating yourself about the contents of certain foods. Once you have a routine going, the time in the kitchen will decrease and your health will improve. But in the beginning you have to keep your discipline up. For example, one thing not allowed on the diet is foods with

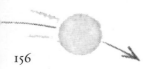

added sugars. When I began reading labels, I found that even most brands of salt had dextrose added to them.

Over years of IBD, the time spent at doctor appointments, pharmacy visits, and possible trips to the hospital will eclipse the cost of using the diet in terms of time and stress as well as dollars. The added boon of fewer visits to the doctor is less interaction with your health insurance company. Unless you're a lover of phone menus and muzak, the less contact with insurance companies, the better.

3. Research note (2002)

The first chapters of *Breaking the Vicious Cycle* discuss the scientific basis for the diet: how IBD, celiac, and diverticulitis patients cannot properly digest many carbohydrates which leads to worsening health. The discussion mentions a synthetic "elemental diet" which has been successfully used for IBD patients. The CCFA Research News Bulletin for Fall 2002 mentions the results of the latest elemental diet study. In two clinical trials with a total of 81 children with Crohn's disease, elemental nutritional therapy showed "a more rapid effect than steroids in inducing clinical remission, and may also heal the intestinal lining (known as the mucosa), which has been damaged by inflammation." Remission was achieved in 90% of the children (CCFA *Under the Microscope* ...4).

The elemental diet has a major drawback in that it's usually administered through a tube inserted into either the stomach or nose – it isn't a sustainable way to live. However, it's similar to the SCD in that the principal carbohydrate is glucose – a monosaccharide that doesn't have to be broken down further before it is absorbed by the body. The underlying rationale for the SCD – eat only what the body can digest – is the same as the elemental diet therapy.

4. Research note (2009)

In recent years, Gottschall's premise of intestinal bacteria playing a role in IBD has gained acceptance. Below is a quote from a *New England Journal of Medicine* article on Inflammatory Bowel Disease printed on August 8, 2002:

> Accumulating evidence suggests that the luminal flora is a requisite and perhaps central factor in the development of inflam-

matory bowel disease. (Podolsky 418)

[Note: "luminal flora" is "intestinal bacteria".]

Since the 2002 article above, medical journals have published dozens of studies regarding bacteria that can benefit the body, better known as probiotics. Certain strains of probiotics have been shown to keep ulcerative colitis in remission longer (Sheil, Shanahan, and O'Mahony 821S), repair the intestinal wall (Resta-Lenert and Barrett 175), and signal intestinal cells to decrease inflammation caused by Crohn's disease (N Borruel, et al. 659).

However, of the many types of probiotics, few have been studied. For example, lactobacillus acidophilus, found in most yogurt made from cow's milk, has been shown to improve the functioning of the intestine. However, in 2008, scientists knew of 144 other species of lactobacillus, in addition to lactobacillus acidophilus (Claesson, van Sinderen, and O'Toole 2945). Ongoing probiotic research promises to deliver tools to better help manage IBD.

Compared to probiotics alone, the SCD uses a two-part approach:

1. Avoiding foods that feed harmful bacteria and cannot be digested when your intestine is injured.

2. Helping restore the balance of beneficial bacteria by using probiotics, particularly in the form of homemade yogurt.

Note: Many probiotic supplements are untested and contain additional strains of bacteria that may or may not be beneficial for certain conditions. If you plan to use a probiotic supplement, talk to your doctor or another reputable source regarding the strains of bacteria as well as trusted brands.

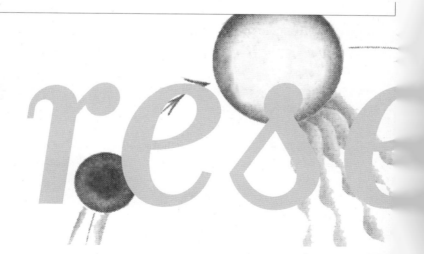

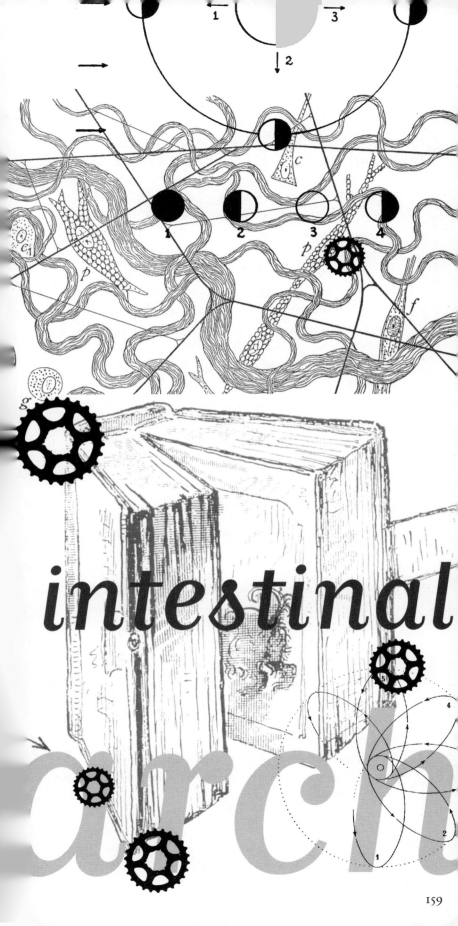

intestinal

arch

ATTITUDE NOW

Since my ulcerative colitis diagnosis, my attitude toward the "traditional" medical establishment has undergone many shifts. At the end of my junior year of high school I had completed classes in Chemistry, Anatomy & Physiology, and Advanced Placement Biology – considered a college level course. These classes built up my respect for the sciences and how this knowledge may be used to improve health.

After being diagnosed with ulcerative colitis, the classes gave me enough background to navigate through medical articles and books written about the disease. If the articles agreed on nothing else, they all said inflammatory bowel disease had no cure and no medication had proven to bring about sustained remission. In addition to these hopeless forecasts, my high school experiences, especially when I was simultaneously taking prednisone, coedine, and donnatal, soured my view of doctors and science in general. I didn't want to know anything else about science. After weaning off the prednisone before college, I dumped all of my pills into the pond near my house. (Even now there may be a bloated, osteoporotic, psychotic bass full of prednisone swimming at high speeds for no reason.)

But in the following months, after discarding the meds, I needed to buy new ones: I went back on Azulfidine, used Pentasa for a brief period, and was introduced to Rowasa enemas. Halfway through college, probably to my detriment, I went off all medications. Azulfidine and Pentasa didn't seem to help much and if my body was going to self-destruct, I didn't want to lose my mind at the same time by taking prednisone.

When I decided to start the diet, I had come out of the hospital for the third time and in the condition I wanted to avoid: prednisone coursed through my veins. The book, *Breaking the Vicious Cycle*, states that you should work with your doctor when using the SCD diet and that you should gradually taper off medication as symptoms clear up. I tapered off the prednisone, stayed on the diet, and here I am: healthy.

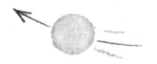

Now my attitude has shifted again. I again respect medication in its power but am aware of its limitations. Medication has a place in acute situations but when used over the long term for IBD, it does not get to the root of the problem and brings along a host of side effects.

Since starting the SCD I have traveled out of the country on numerous occasions, including seven to India. For most of the trips I brought along "emergency" prednisone and returned with the seals on the bottles unbroken. However, for one trip, feeling untouchable, I failed to take back-up medication, and, after eating at a restaurant, fell ill from food poisoning. I spent days either kneeling on the cool tiles by a commode or sitting on it. I failed to keep down food or water. When I returned home I spent several days in the hospital. Medication knocked back the flare-up and the diet kept the remission going. Because I knew what to expect, recovery came with relative ease and I have traveled again, with the pill bottle unopened.

For my long term health, I follow the diet to keep IBD in remission. However, if another unexpected situation arises, I will use medication to arrest an acute situation.

+ ◈ + ◈ + ◈ + ◈

My wife and I bought a house in 2002 and I've spent hours stripping and refinishing old molding and doors, painting, building bookshelves and a bed, cutting down a dying tree, cleaning twenty years of dust out of the basement, and other things that come along with property ownership. I've been feeling good when I'm working, even springy. Reading back on this journal-turned-into-short-book, I'm happy to be healthy and strong. I'm a changed person. It didn't take much: Not having to arrange my day based on bathroom location, not taking medication, being "regular," and having much more energy were enough.

If I could re-do my first eight years with ulcerative colitis, I would start by reading and getting more information on the Specfic Carbohydrate Diet.

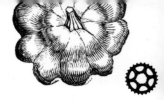

Below are some places to begin:

> (book): Your primary source on the diet should be the book *Breaking the Vicious Cycle* by Elaine Gottschall. Check your library, bookstore, or online vendors such as amazon.com.

> (websites):
www.breakingtheviciouscycle.info
www.scdrecipe.com
www.lucyskitchenshop.com
www.scdiet.org
www.pecanbread.com
www.digestivewellness.com
www.scdiet.net
www.scdbakery.com
www.gottschallcenter.com

Before closing I want to thank Elaine Gottschall for writing her book. I first met her in 2001, at an SCD brunch in Long Island. I had seen her photo in the back of the book as well as on a website – a kind grandmotherly face. As I made my way to the back of the restaurant with a view of docks and the Long Island Sound beyond, I imagined her as a warm, soft-spoken woman. She is warm and kind, but at 5'8" and with as much energy as people decades younger, she knocked me out with her knowledge and the story of how she came to write the book. In a time when turning on the news sends you scurrying, her story is enough to get you going again:

Elaine's daughter Judy was diagnosed with a severe case of ulcerative colitis at the age of four and a half. By the age of eight, despite years of treatment with cortisone and sulfonamides, Judy's condition deteriorated. Upon examination, over a dozen doctors said that her intestines would have to be removed. Almost out of hope, Elaine and her husband brought their daughter to Dr. Haas, an elderly pediatrician whom the *New York Times* described as a "pioneer in pediatrics." Dr. Haas recommended what is now known as the Specific Carbohydrate Diet. Within one year on the diet, Judy had been weaned off all medications and returned to full strength. From that time until now, Judy continues to live a healthy life while following the SCD. However, Elaine became increasingly frustrated

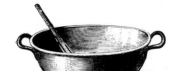

as she heard of friends and acquaintances with IBD who underwent experiences with prednisone and surgery. In these situations she would relate her daughter's experiences with the diet. However, she could not recommend any scientists or health professionals who would or could describe the science behind the diet, and, unfortunately, Dr. Haas had passed away at the age of 94.

Taking it upon herself to help IBD sufferers, Elaine returned to school to learn why the diet worked. Not having taken a class since 1939, she returned to high school at the age of 45 to brush up on math. After completing this step, Elaine realized that to continue undergraduate and graduate studies would take many years. However, she did not deviate from her goal and spent ten years in universities: First at Montclair State College in New Jersey, where she received her bachelor's degree in 1973, graduating Magna Cum Laude. From there, she spent a year in the Department of Graduate Studies in Nutrition at Rutgers, The State University of New Jersey.

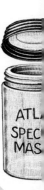

In 1975, she became a member of the Department of Cell Science at The University of Western Ontario's Zoology Department and spent four years there investigating the effects of various sugars on the digestive tract. She obtained a Master of Science degree in that Department in 1979. Results of her work are published in the Journal, *Acta Anatomica* 123: 178 (1985). For the year following, Elaine worked in the Department of Anatomy of the University of Western Ontario investigating the changes that occur in the bowel wall in inflammatory bowel disease.

In 1987, she completed work on a book titled *Food and the Gut Reaction.* In it she described the mechanisms which perpetuate IBD and how to use diet to wean off medication and return the body to a healthy state. While the first half of the book explained the biology and chemistry behind the diet, the second half contained recipes. Ms. Gottschall and her husband, who gave his wholehearted support to her endeavors, self-published the book. In two years, it barely sold 200 copies. However, Ms. Gottschall, by then a Canadian resident, continued to speak vigorously about the diet and was invited to appear on Dina Petty, the Canadian version of Oprah Winfrey. Elaine's segment ran for 8 minutes on national TV. In the next 10 days 23,000 copies of the book were sold and word began to spread. In 1994, she re-published the book

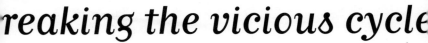

reaking the vicious cycle

under the name *Breaking the Vicious Cycle*. Currently in its eighth printing, the book has sold over 3 million copies. Her house contains a collection of thousands of thank-you notes from people who use the diet to control IBD as well as countless e-mails.

Elaine Gottschall passed away on September 5, 2005, at her home in Canada. We will all miss her lively fighting spirit.

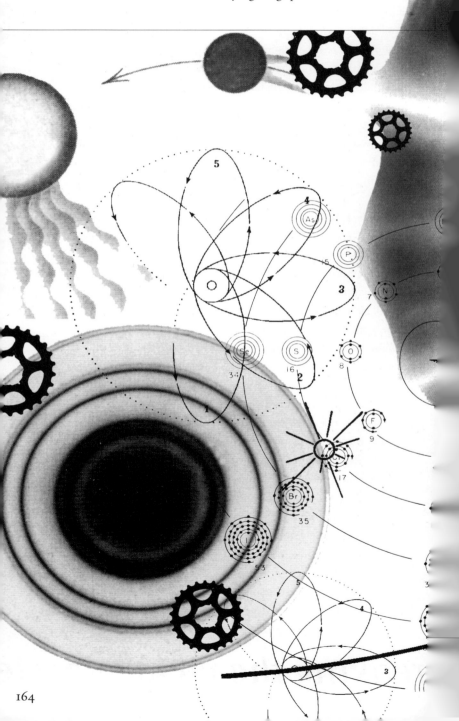

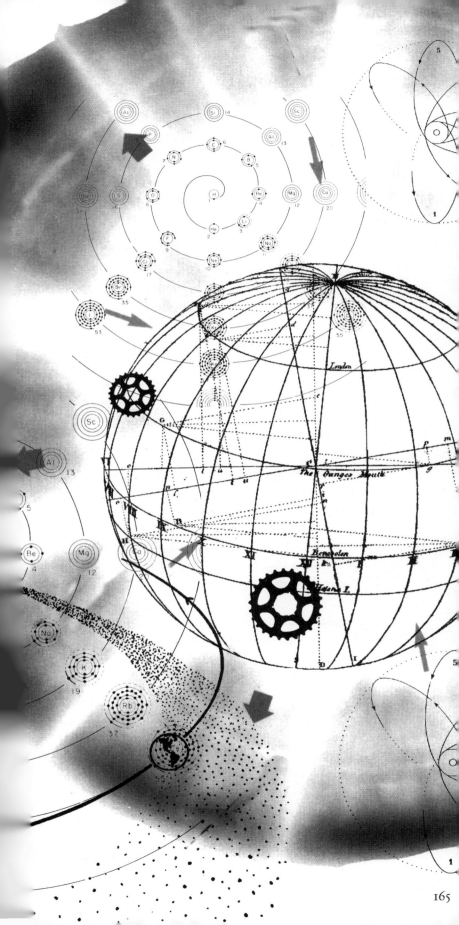

WORKS CITED

Baker, Don. "Once a stepchild, P&G's drug business grows up." **The Cinncinati Post**. n. pag. Online. Internet. 19 Apr. 2002. Available http://www.cincypost.com/2002/apr/20/pg04 2002.html.

Barrett, Amy. "Johnson & Johnson: A Shopping Spree Waiting to Happen." **Business Week Online**. n. pag. Online. Internet. 17 Jun. 2002. Available http://www.businessweek.com.

Borruel, N. et al. "Increased mucosal tumour necrosis factor α production in Crohn's disease can be downregulated ex vivo by probiotic bacteria." **Gut** 2002; 51:659–664

Claesson, Marcus J., Douwe van Sinderen and Paul W. O'Toole. "Lactobacillus phylogenomics – towards a reclassification of the genus." **International Journal of Systematic and Evolutionary Microbiology** 2008; 58: 2945–2954

Crohn's & Colitis Foundation of America. **Crohn's Disease & Ulcerative Colitis: Surgery.** New York: Crohn's & Colitis Foundation of America, 2002.

Crohn's & Colitis Foundation of America. **Crohn's Disease & Ulcerative Colitis: Understanding Colorectal Cancer.** New York: Crohn's & Colitis Foundation of America, 2002.

Crohn's & Colitis Foundation of America. **Under the Microscope: Research News Bulletin from the Crohn's & Colitis Foundation of America.** Fall 2002.

Fiondella, Francesco. "Eating is Believing: Patients Suffering from Crohn's disease say diet can help their pain. But doctors ask: Show us the proof." **Wall Street Journal.** 11 Nov 2002: R6, R11.

Medical Economics Staff. **Physicians' Desk Reference 2002.** Montvale: Medical Economics Company, Inc., 2002.

Podolsky, Daniel K. "Inflammatory Bowel Disease." **New England Journal of Medicine** 2002 Aug 8; 347(6):417-29

Resta-Lenert, Silvia C. and Kim E. Barrett. "Modulation of Intestinal Barrier Properties by Probiotics: Role in Reversing Colitis." **Annals of the New York Academy of Sciences** 2009; 1165:175-182

Sheil, Barbara, Fergus Shanahan, and Liam O'Mahony. "Probiotic Effects on Inflammatory Bowel Disease." **The Journal of Nutrition** 2007; 137:819S–824S

WebMD Inc. "Infliximab [brand name: Remicade]." **WebMD_Health**. n. pag. Online. Internet. 11 Nov 2002. Available http://my.webmd.com/content/drugs/3/4046-6306

WebMD Inc. "Prednisone." **WebMD_Health**. n. pag. Online. Internet. 11 Nov 2002. Available http://my.webmd.com/content/drugs/2/4046-1741

Zonderman, Jon and Ronald Vender, M.D. **Understanding Ulcerative Colitis & Crohn Disease**. Jackson: University Press of Mississippi, 2000.

NOTES

[1] Two examples of the "hundreds of millions of dollars" spent on IBD are Asacol with recent revenues of approximately $300 million and Remicade with $721 million. These figures are from **The Cinncinati Post** and **Business Week Online**, respectively.

IMAGE SOURCES

All of the medical graphics came from the book **Images of Medicine: A Definitive Volume of More Than 4,800 Copyright-Free Engravings Including Anatomy, General Medicine, Apothecary and Pharmaceuti** by Jim Harter (Editor). Published: New York: Bonanza Books, 1991.

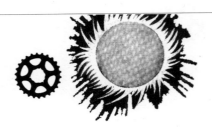

ACKNOWLEDGEMENTS

I want to thank my family and friends for supporting this project. Particularly, the graphic designer N. who made every page a visual treat.

The names of doctors, the good and the bad, have been changed as have the names of medical facilities.

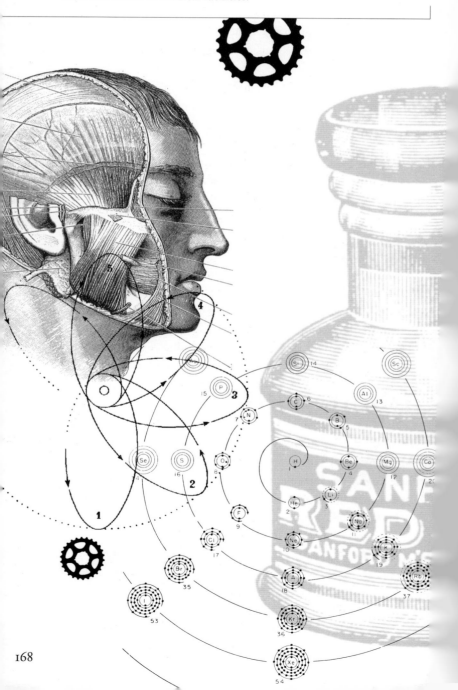

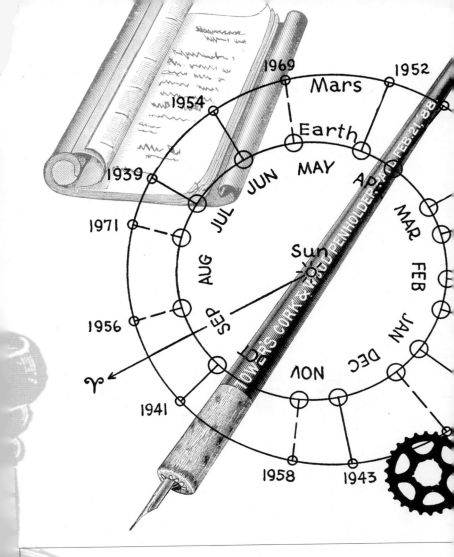

ABOUT THE AUTHOR

The author currently lives in a house with a blue-green study, a yellow-orange chair, a black-white dog, and his designer wife in Boston, MA. This is his first (and last) book about his intestines. He regained his health from critical investigations in libraries, bookstores, and the internet. He maintains the SCDRecipe.com website which contains a compilation of recipes for the SCD community. In 2004, he published a cookbook called "Adventures in the Family Kitchen." His third book "Recipes for the Specific Carbohydrate Diet" was released by Fair Winds Press in 2008.

The author grew up in North Haven, Connecticut. He received his B.S. from Cornell in 1994, and M.Sc. from Rensselaer Polytechnic Institute in 1999.

DESIGN & PRINTING

DESIGN:
Niloufer Moochhala / NYMDesign
www.nymdesign.com

PRINTING:
JAK Printers
Mumbai (Bombay), India

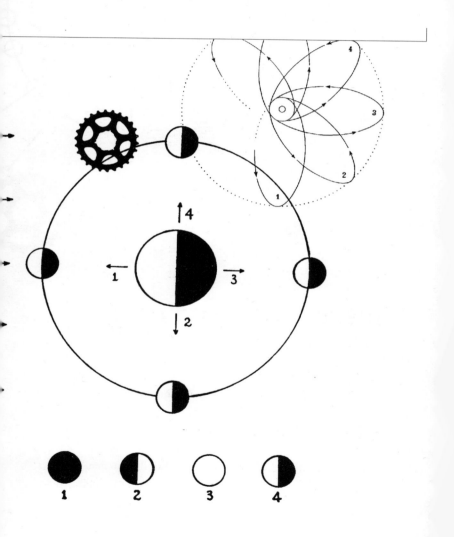

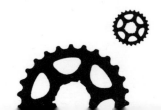